LEGS UP!

The Ultimate Troubleshooting Guide for Your Vagina

by
GAIL S. KING, MD

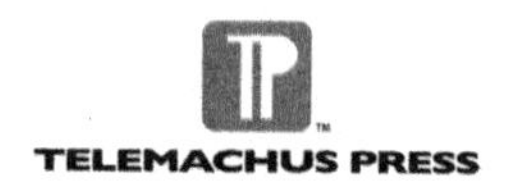
TELEMACHUS PRESS

LEGS UP! The Ultimate Troubleshooting Guide for Your Vagina

Cover designed by Telemachus Press, LLC

The author acknowledges permission from Reckonwith Enterprises to reprint quote by Amanda Reckon.

Published by Telemachus Press, LLC
http://www.telemachuspress.com

Visit the author website:
http://www.DrGailKing.com

ISBN: 978-1-940745-65-7 (eBook)
ISBN: 978-1-940745-66-4 (Paperback)

Version 2014.12.14

Printed in the United States of America
10 9 8 7 6 5 4 3 2 1 0

Disclaimer

The information and ideas in this book reflect the medical training and clinical experience of the author. Every attempt has been made to present accurate, state-of-the-art material. Not all the information, statements, advice, opinions, or suggestions set forth in the material contained in this book have been evaluated by the FDA and should not be relied upon to diagnose, treat, cure, or prevent any condition or disease.

The information provided is for general reference purposes only, and is not intended to replace individual evaluation and treatment by your physician or other qualified healthcare professionals. Each woman's health needs, risks, and goals are different and should be developed with medical supervision for personalized advice, answers to specific medical questions, and individual recommendations. If you have specific medical symptoms, consult your physician immediately. Discuss any recommendations in this book with your physician to determine if he or she has a different perspective.

Product trademark names are used throughout this book to describe or inform the reader about the various proprietary products that are owned by others. The presentation of such information is intended to benefit the owners of the products and trademarks and is not intended to infringe upon trademark, copyright or other rights, nor to imply or make a claim other than those claims made by the owners. The owners of such products and trademarks have given no endorsement of the information in this book, and the inclusion of product trademarks in this book does not imply endorsement.

This book is dedicated to all my current and future patients.

Together, we're making Aspen more beautiful, one vagina at a time.

Gail S. King MD

Men are told to grow a pair,
Get some balls,
Hang 'em there.
Women take the greater hits,
They're equipped with catcher's mitts.

Amanda Reckon

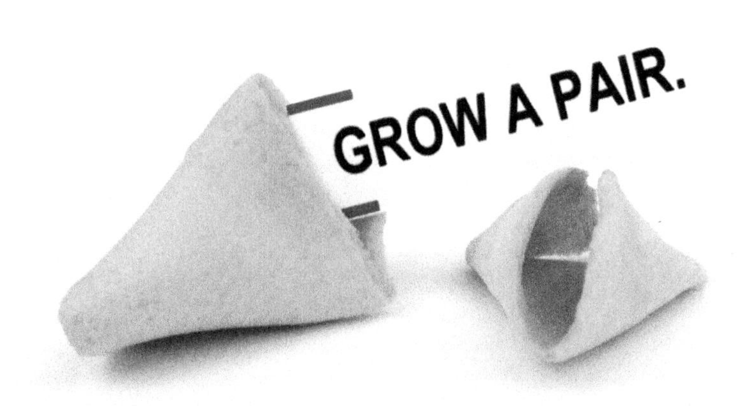

Contents

Introduction

Vaginas. Every woman has one.

Nature designed it well; after all, your reproductive system is the key to survival of our human species.

Your vagina is a little tube, usually about three to seven inches long, that connects the outside world to the end of your uterus. When it's working as nature intended, your vagina will be tight enough to enclose and stimulate an erect penis, but also supple and stretchy enough to provide safe passage for your newborn baby as it enters this world.

Over the course of your lifetime, from puberty to old age, your vagina endures all manner of stress and strain, causing problems that need to be corrected before they turn into major disasters. I've coined a term for these problems: Vagina Dilemmas. Now who would have thought that one little body part could be the source of so many Dilemmas?

Along the way in this book, we'll meet some Granny Vagina Dilemmas. The term Granny Vagina does not refer to your age—far from it. Granny Vagina is my term for describing the way a young woman's vaginal tissue looks if it becomes weak, dry, or thin, like that of an eighty-year-old woman. You certainly don't need to be old enough to be a granny in order for you to have Granny Vagina Dilemmas.

This book has been inspired by women patients who have come in to see me over the course of my practice. Many of my patients have no vaginal problems, and I am happy to send them on their way with a clean bill of health after I've finished their pelvic exams. Then there are some patients who already have an inkling of impending trouble with their lady-parts. And others who are outright horrified by symptoms they are experiencing down there.

I am concerned that so many women don't know what's happening inside their vaginas, causing their problems. And what's more, there has been no place to go to learn about Vagina Dilemmas in detail. It's certainly not something you would have learned about early in life; it's not covered in school sex education classes, not even in Biology. In our society, vaginal issues have traditionally been an undignified topic, something taboo that we don't talk about.

Although an estimated thirty-four million women worldwide are affected by prolapse (when one of the body organs drops out of its natural place inside the pelvic area), and millions more suffer sexual dysfunction that originates in the vagina, women are reluctant to discuss vaginal issues, even with their doctor. This reluctance has resulted in a great silence; many women today are simply unaware that they do not have to live with the pain and trauma that plagued their mothers and grandmothers.

Women today do not have to live with the pain and trauma that plagued their mothers and grandmothers.

In my practice, I often have to encourage patients to talk about their vaginas. During a pelvic examination when I ask a patient if she is experiencing any problems, it's not unusual to get one of three standard answers: Either my patient doesn't know that her symptoms indicate her vaginal tissue is dangerously weak and thin. Or she suspects something serious but doesn't know how to talk about it. Or she takes her problem for granted—she thinks her symptoms are something she just has to live with because "that's what happens to women."

If I prod further and ask my patient, for example, if she leaks urine, a typical response might be, "Not that bad." Or, "It doesn't happen very often." When I inquire whether sex is tight enough for her, she might say, "It's fine," when it isn't fine at all. Or, "It never occurred to me it should be tighter." These problems are Vagina Dilemmas that shouldn't be ignored.

So, I decided to write a patient-friendly book about this serious subject. (After all, what could be more serious to you than what's going on in the vicinity of your vagina?) When I told one of my patients about it she said, "Dr. King, don't make my eyes glaze over with twelve-letter-long medical terms." Don't worry, I won't. I didn't write this book in a manner suitable for a scholarly medical journal. Instead, I wrote this book in the friendly language that I use to explain Vagina Dilemmas to my patients every single day.

My intent is to present an easy-to-read reference that is simple enough to understand, but also specific enough to give you a clear idea of your Vagina Dilemma symptoms, as well as their implications. With that in mind, I trust you'll find this book to be light, enjoyable and educational.

You have the power to become an informed patient—to know what's normal, what's not normal, and to take greater control of changes to your vagina over time. Use this book as a base from which to have questions ready that you want answered when you are with your doctor.

For those of you who still feel a bit shy about this aspect of your body, I trust that, after reading this book, you'll become increasingly comfortable with your sexuality. And remember, this book is designed to be your personal resource. Keep a copy tucked in the drawer with your undies; refer to it over time as your body ages and you experience different aspects of Vagina Dilemmas.

No matter what condition your vagina is in, nobody wants a Granny Vagina!

Part

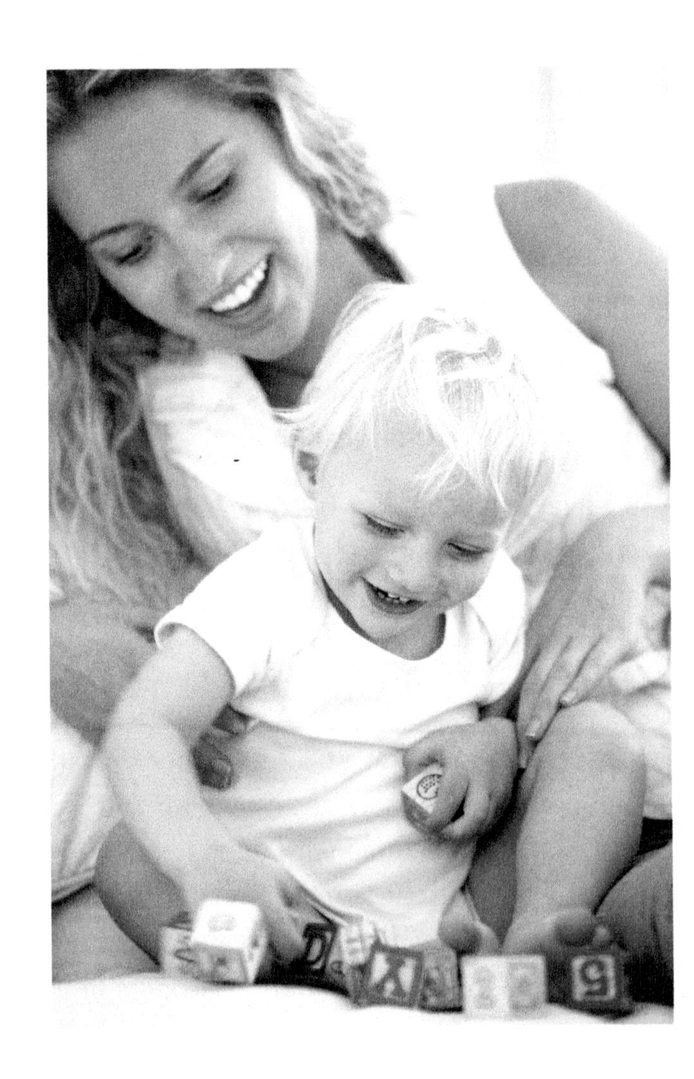

One

Your Young Vagina

Chapter One

Legs Up! Now Hold That Pose

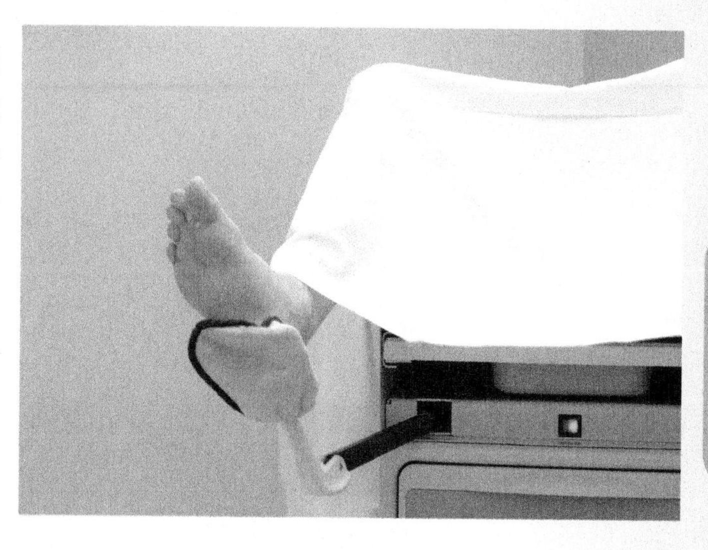

There you are, splayed out on my exam table, feet up in the stirrups, your bare bottom catching the breeze under the big white sheet. "Just my annual exam," you think.

You wonder if you should bring up that problem you've always been reluctant to admit to anyone. Or those signs you've noticed that something might not be quite right down there. "No," you rationalize. "It's probably nothing. And besides, it's all too embarrassing to talk about."

Little do you realize that your embarrassment could be leading you into big trouble.

Your embarrassment could be leading you into big trouble.

But you try to stare nonchalantly at the ceiling while I adjust my light and take a look at what you're presenting. **"Oh my," you hear me exclaim. "You've got a Granny Vagina!"**

An image of a wizened old grandmother in a rocking chair pops into your head. "Granny Vagina? Surely not me," you protest.

"I'm nowhere near being a granny. I'm still young."

"Well," I continue, "your vagina looks eighty years old."

You're mortified. Whatever your Granny Vagina is, you want to pull the sheet right up over your head—shield yourself from prying eyes.

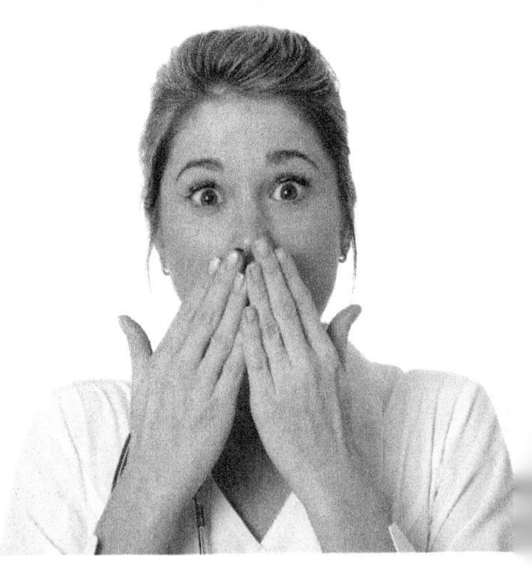

"That's horrible," you think. "What's going on down there?"

"Tell me, Doctor," you whisper. "Is it bad? What's the worst thing that could happen to me?"

The Worst Thing That Could Happen

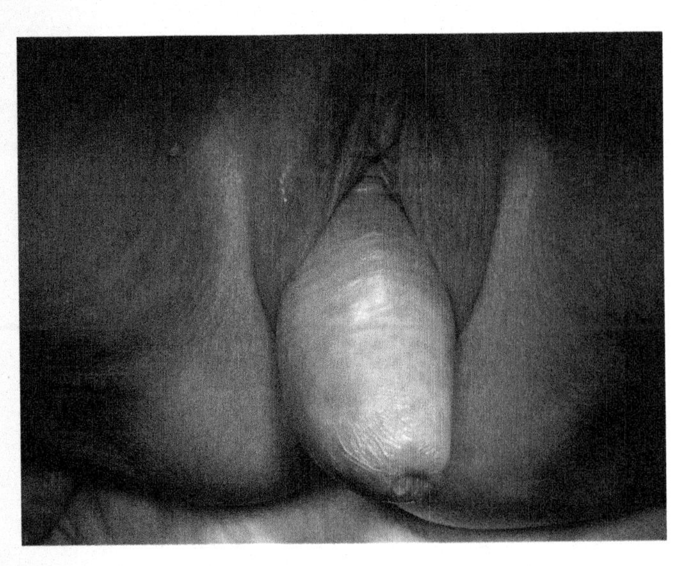

"Oh my God!"

"That's GROSS!"

"Is this a real picture?"

"Is this what's going to happen to me?"

Procidentia (Uterine Prolapse)

Granny Vagina: What Does It Mean?

You started out with what nature gave you: your vaginal opening was tight. Inside, your vaginal area was pink and plump; your tissue was thick; it was moist and had elasticity; it had folds (rugations).

I've coined the term "Granny Vagina" to mean a vagina (no matter what your age) that doesn't look young, healthy, taunt, or tight anymore. Having a Granny Vagina does not mean you are old—far from it. When you are still young, something can be going on inside your vagina to give it characteristics typically found in old women.

Granny Vagina Disaster

This picture shows you the worst instance of Granny Vagina. If you think about what can happen in the vagina as "shades of gray," this shade is black.

This tragedy is what happens when you wait until it's too late.

I call this stage DISASTER.

Yes, it's a real picture (unretouched) of a patient I had not seen before in my office. She called one morning in a state of panic. (Wouldn't you be?) The tissue holding her uterus in place had become so thin that it allowed her uterus to "come loose from its moorings" and fall. What you are looking at is her uterus after it fell down through her vaginal canal. Because her vagina had become baggy and badly stretched out, her runaway uterus poked right through to the outside.

Don't wait for Granny Vagina Disaster to happen.

I took this picture just before I started surgery to put this lady's uterus back up inside her body cavity and tack it in place so that it wouldn't come falling out again.

"Why didn't anyone ever tell me?"

"It's not my fault I have a Granny Vagina, Dr. King," you say defensively. "I take good care of my health. I have always gone for my routine check-up. Every year. And they've always done a pelvic exam.

"No one's told me before I had something going on down there. Why didn't anyone ever tell me?"

That's an important question. Later in this book, I devote a whole chapter to "Why Didn't Anyone Ever Tell Me?" The answer may surprise you!

All Those Terms

I promise this book will be easy to read: I purposefully avoid using technical jargon. As we come across medical terms, I'll explain each one in context, along with a short definition. You'll also find a glossary of terms at the end of the book.

Coming to Terms

Here's a term you'll be seeing many times in the following chapters: ***prolapse***. Prolapse means "to drop" or "to sink."

Whenever one of your body organs drops out of its natural place inside your pelvic area, we say it has prolapsed.

Coming to Terms

As the name indicates, uterine prolapse happens when your uterus drops down into your vagina. The medical term is ***procidentia***.

Nobody Wants a Granny Vagina

When I examine the muscles, ligaments and supporting tissue inside a woman's vaginal area, I look for signs that these supports have become weakened and less able to hold organs (such as her uterus) in place. Over the course of a lifetime, as many as one in eight women will suffer prolapse of the uterus to some degree.

Seek medical attention to have your Granny Vagina fixed.

As you progress through this book, you'll learn to identify the most common instances of Granny Vagina. If you find yourself in these pages, you need to seek medical attention so that your Granny Vagina can be fixed before it's too late.

In the next chapter, "Disaster Happens: Prolapsed Uterus," we'll explore this Granny Vagina Disaster further.

Chapter Two

Disaster Happens: Prolapsed Uterus

Granny Vagina Disaster: "OMG! Something's hanging out!"

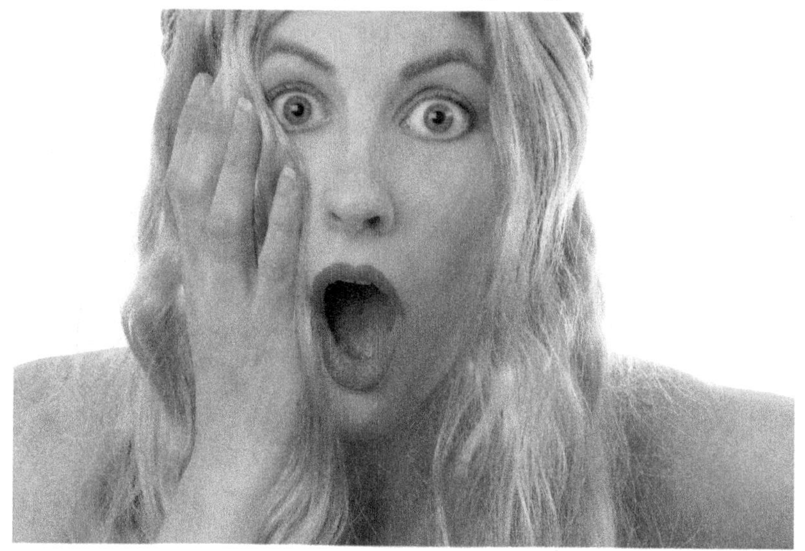

I've chosen to start with the worst thing that could happen to you, because I want to stress the **urgency of not waiting too long to have your Granny Vagina problems corrected.**

Your vaginal problems might start out small, but if your vaginal tissue is thinning, and you wait so long that it becomes too weak to hold your uterus in place, your uterus may come falling out. Just like you saw in our picture from the last chapter.

Yes, Prolapsed Uterus Could Happen to You

Don't think, "It won't happen to me." If your pelvic muscles and ligaments are too weak to hold your uterus in place, and you wait until it's too late, all it will take is something stressful to tip your uterus over the edge. It can happen suddenly.

Don't think, "It won't happen to me."

Maybe you'll be out running. (Can you imagine how scary it would be to have your uterus fall and come bulging through your vagina while you're out on the trail, far from help?)

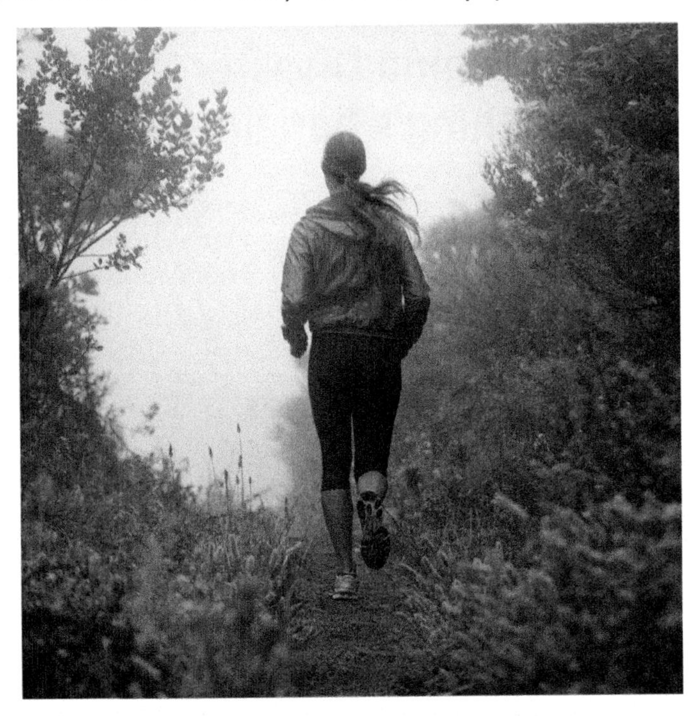

Or your uterus could fall because you have a cold and you've been coughing for weeks. One strong cough and POP, out it flies! It's frightening, like a hernia poking through. Here are some examples of stress factors leading to prolapsed uterus:

- Running or jogging
- Exercising

- Bad cough
- Heavy lifting
- Being overweight
- Giving birth vaginally
- Prior surgery
- Chronic constipation

A few other factors may also play a part in weakening your pelvic muscles and ligaments; for example, researchers are studying the effects of ethnicity and genetics.

Elderly Ladies Are at Risk

Granted, it's not uncommon for an elderly lady in frail health to develop a prolapsed uterus. Maybe you've heard of an older woman in your family who had a "fallen uterus." Perhaps she was in a nursing home, bedridden, unable to tolerate surgery, so that securing her uterus back in place was not an option. Usually, in these cases the nurses just push her uterus back up and keep her in diapers. Not a pleasant thought, is it?

This Disaster's Not Just for Old Ladies

But we're talking about you. You've not even reached menopause, and already you could be at risk for a prolapsed uterus.

Case in Point

The lady in our picture wasn't that old. She was only in her forties, had several children, and she hadn't gone through menopause yet. Tragically, no one had warned her about the signs of her impending Granny Vagina Disaster.

It Needn't Happen to You

*Although a prolapsed uterus is the worst Granny Vagina Disaster that **could happen** to you, it **needn't happen** to you.*

Are There Warning Signs?

Yes, there are warning signs to indicate your uterus is in danger of coming unhitched. And these signs should never be ignored. Symptoms depend on how severe the prolapse is.

Many times, patients suffering from a prolapsed uterus admit they had felt something before their uterus gave way. Symptoms you may experience that are common to pelvic organ prolapse include the following:

- A bulge of tissue or lump, often red and sore, may develop in your genital area.
- You may notice a pulling or stretching in your groin area.
- You may develop pain in your pelvis or lower back.
- You may experience vaginal pain, pressure or irritation.
- You may see vaginal discharge, spotting or bleeding.
- Your vagina may come protruding out from your body.
- You may experience delayed or slow urinary stream or ***urinary incontinence*** (losing control of your bladder).
- You may have difficulty with bowel movements or ***fecal incontinence*** (losing control of your bowel).
- You may experience sexual problems, including decreased sex drive.
- Sexual intercourse may become difficult or painful.

Degrees of Impending Disaster

A careful and thorough pelvic examination is essential for identifying the presence and severity of vaginal prolapse.

During your exam, a stage from zero to four will be assigned, based on what the exam shows:

- Stage 0—no prolapse present
- Stage I—a bulge that comes down into the top one-third of the vagina
- Stage II—protrusion one-third to two-thirds down the vaginal canal
- Stage III—protrusion into the bottom one-third of the vagina
- Stage IV—the organ or vaginal wall protrudes through the opening

Patients with **Stage 0** or **Stage I** prolapse are not presently at risk.

When I examine a patient, I may find that her uterus has prolapsed into her vaginal canal. The descriptive term for this condition is **Stage II or Second Degree**. If her signs indicate that her uterus has not come down very far, she may not be at risk of it giving way just then. With Second Degree, we're going to watch her condition every single year. I instruct this patient: "If you start losing urine, having pain or other trouble, you should get in here right away."

When a woman's uterus definitely drops, her prolapse has progressed to **Stage III or Third Degree.** Often, her ***urethra*** (the tube that carries urine out of the body) becomes kinked so that she has trouble passing urine. I tell this patient: "Don't wait. Be fixed now. If you suffer and wait until it gets awful—and it will—your condition will progress to DISASTER!"

Stage IV or Fourth Degree simply means DISASTER. The uterus has come sliding out—like it did with the lady in our picture. For the patient whose uterus hangs entirely out of her vagina, there is only one choice for repair: surgery.

Granny Vagina Dilemma: "But I don't see any trouble brewing down there."

Except in the most advanced cases of prolapse, you probably won't be able to see trouble brewing down there in your lady-parts. Because your reproductive organs are so important, Mother Nature hid much of your female sexual apparatus up inside you (unlike men, who carry their genitals around outside their bodies, where they are easier to see).

Interestingly, there's a lot going on inside you, especially in your lower abdomen. As we move through the following chapters, you can refer to the Appendix for descriptions of the organs inside your pelvis that contribute to various Granny Vagina Dilemmas, as well as pictures of how they all fit together.

Men carry their genitals around outside their bodies, where they are easier to see.

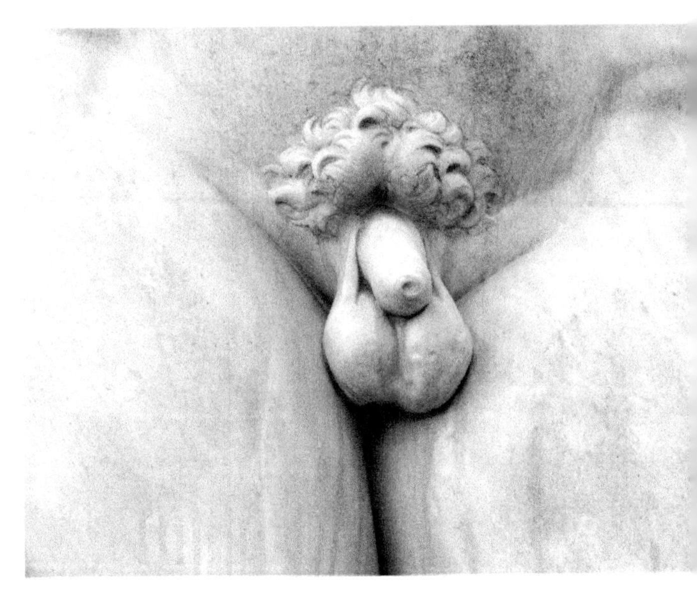

Looking Ahead

There's trouble ahead if the muscles, tissue and ligaments that are intended to support your pelvic organs in their rightful place become weak, torn or stretched. Then, the organs may sag downward. As they drop, they push against or into your vagina (referred to as ***pelvic organ prolapse*** or ***pelvic support defects***).

In the next chapter, which I have labeled "Other Organs Falling Down," we'll look at other serious Granny Vagina Dilemmas that can occur down there in the region of your female sex apparatus.

Chapter Three

Other Organs Falling Down

Now that I've caught your attention with the scary Granny Vagina Disaster (that prolapsed uterus of the last chapter), let's assume you have come in to see me because something is amiss down there. After we've talked a bit and you feel comfortable enough to let your guard down, it's time for you to confess: you're curious about some embarrassing, out-of-the-ordinary symptoms you've noticed. You might be blissfully unaware, however, that certain signs you are experiencing point to impending trouble.

Really Embarrassing

Let's start with one of the most embarrassing Dilemmas you can endure: bladder prolapse, which is what happens when your bladder comes tumbling down.

Granny Vagina Dilemma: "I pee my pants in public."

SYMPTOM: If your bladder begins to push down into your vaginal area, leakage of urine becomes an embarrassing problem. You will lose small or moderate amounts of urine with normal physical activities, such as when you laugh or cough. More strenuous activities—like walking, running, or jumping—cause you to pee involuntarily.

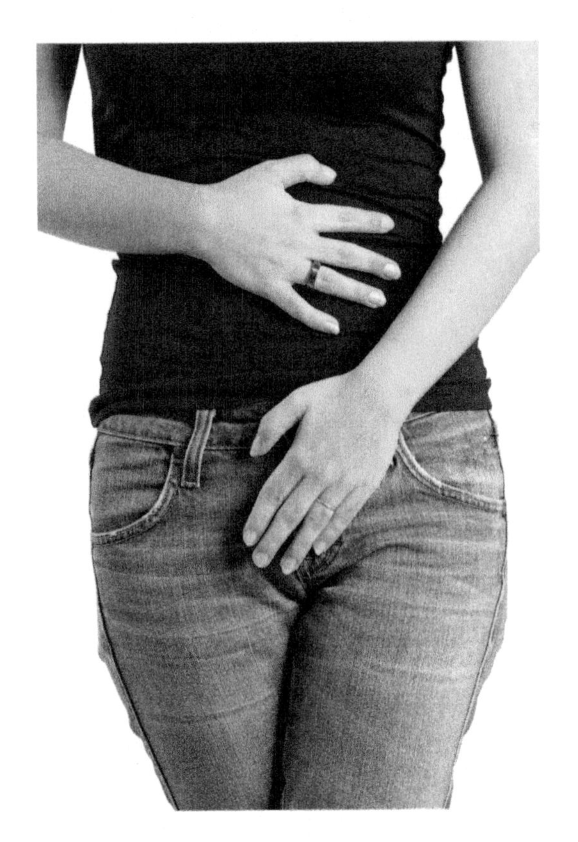

It's No Laughing Matter

You may see tee shirts with what the designers intend to be a "cute" saying: *"Sometimes I laugh so hard tears run down my legs."*

This condition ceases to be funny and turns into a Dilemma when it happens to you. Laughter should be enjoyed, not dreaded. Who wants to sit around with a sour face at a party, just because you're afraid you'll piddle out a puddle if you laugh?

Variations:

- At the gym, I dribble on the treadmill.
- Don't stand near me when I jump or you'll get wet.
- I'm just walking or jogging along—and squirt.

- I pee when I have sex.
- A cough or sneeze is all it takes.
- Lifting is risky.

Coming to Terms

The ability to hold urine in the bladder and control urine flow is ***continence***. Difficulty controlling the start and stop of urine flow, or accidental loss of urine, is ***incontinence***.

A Stressful Situation

Inability to control bursts of urine is ***stress urinary incontinence,*** and just as its name implies, everything may be going along fine until you put a sudden stress on your bladder, causing an increase in abdominal pressure. Then, to your great embarrassment, a spurt of urine escapes. The amount of urine loss may vary from only a few drops to a real catastrophe—enough so that you have to change clothes or wear a pad all the time "just in case."

As many as thirty million American women suffer from symptoms of stress urinary incontinence, making it difficult for them to control spurts of urine in certain situations.

What It's Not

Note that we're not talking here about a continual urge to urinate. You've seen those ads on television about always experiencing an urge to run off to the bathroom to pee. That's urgency incontinence and it's a different problem: there are medications and treatments to help with continual pangs of urgency.

Why Does Stress Urinary Incontinence Happen?

Nature tucked your bladder into its own little space down there in your pelvic area. But the muscles and tissue holding your bladder in place can become weak and give way. When the wall between your bladder and the vagina weakens, your bladder can drop from its normal place and bulge or herniate into the vaginal wall. Then, when a sudden stress on your bladder causes an increase in abdominal pressure, your bladder is squeezed and urine escapes.

Coming to Terms

The medical term for bulging of the bladder into the vagina is ***cystocele***.

A ***cystocele*** occurs when the bladder falls or descends from its normal position. Large cystoceles can cause the bladder to overfill and allow small amounts of urine to leak. Leakage is most common during activity such as walking or bouts of coughing.

Is a Droopy Bladder Always Serious?

Your bladder may drop into the vagina only a little. Such small cystoceles are common. Many women have them and do not experience any urination problems or other symptoms. As long as your bladder drops only a little, you probably don't need surgery to correct it. Pelvic floor exercises, vaginal weights, and biofeedback can often help in mild cases. Whenever I see this stage, I make a note of the condition and keep track of it with every annual pelvic exam. I also tell these patients "If you begin to leak urine or have related symptoms, come in to see me right away."

If your bladder drops farther into your vagina and becomes a hernia that protrudes through the vaginal wall, that's serious.

When this Dilemma happens, you begin leaking urine, your embarrassment starts, and it's time for you to take action. Pelvic surgery can put your bladder back where it belongs and repair the muscle and tissue so that your bladder will be held in its normal place.

When you begin leaking urine, it's time for you to take action.

Just the Opposite

If you thought peeing your pants in public was bad enough, next we'll look at what can happen if you can't pee at all.

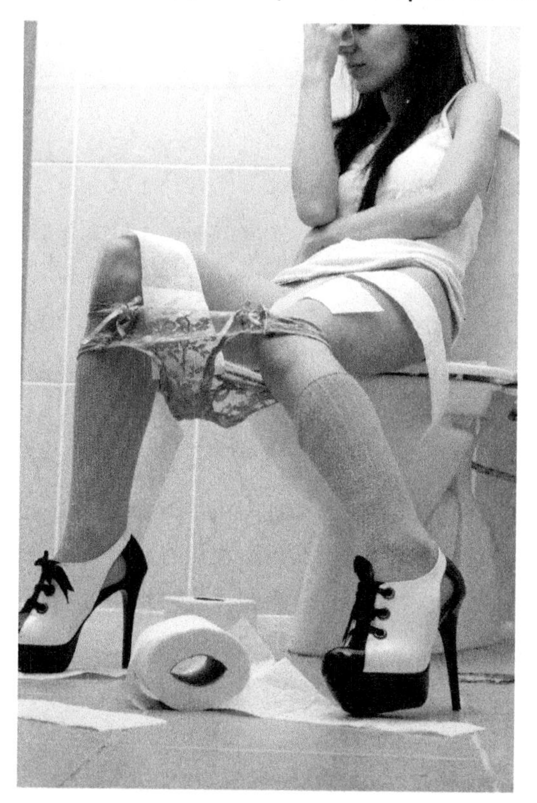

Granny Vagina Dilemma: "I can't wee when I want to."

SYMPTOM: If your bladder drops into a position where it is difficult for urine to pass out of your body, you will begin to notice your urinary stream becomes slow, delayed, or even blocked. You might need to push your bladder back up into the vagina to be able to empty your bladder.

Kinky Problem

It's not uncommon for your ***urethra*** (the little tube that carries urine out of your body) to become kinked when your bladder falls into your vagina. This condition causes problems when you try to pass urine. You will have to strain to push your urine through the kinked-up tube. Some women have to reach back into their vagina and push the bladder out of the way in order to let urine pass.

Coming to Terms

When the urethra bulges into the vaginal wall, it is a ***urethrocele***. A urethrocele usually occurs in conjunction with a cystocele. A ***cystourethrocele*** is a cystocele and urethrocele occurring in combination.

Urine Retention

If your bladder comes loose from its normal place and falls far into your vagina, it might become so displaced that you will be unable to completely empty your bladder. Not only is this condition inconvenient and uncomfortable, but also retaining urine can be a serious medical issue. You should seek gynecological care as soon as possible.

Another Potty Problem

While we're in the area, let's pay a visit to another elimination embarrassment: ***rectal prolapse***. This Dilemma happens when the bowel "pooches up" out of its normal channel and bulges into your vagina.

Coming to Terms

A ***rectal prolapse*** occurs when the bowel "pooches up" out of its normal channel and bulges into your vagina.

Granny Vagina Dilemma: "I've got shitty on my shirttail."

SYMPTOM: If it's your bowel that pops out of place, you may lose control of bowel function, as if it has a mind of its own.

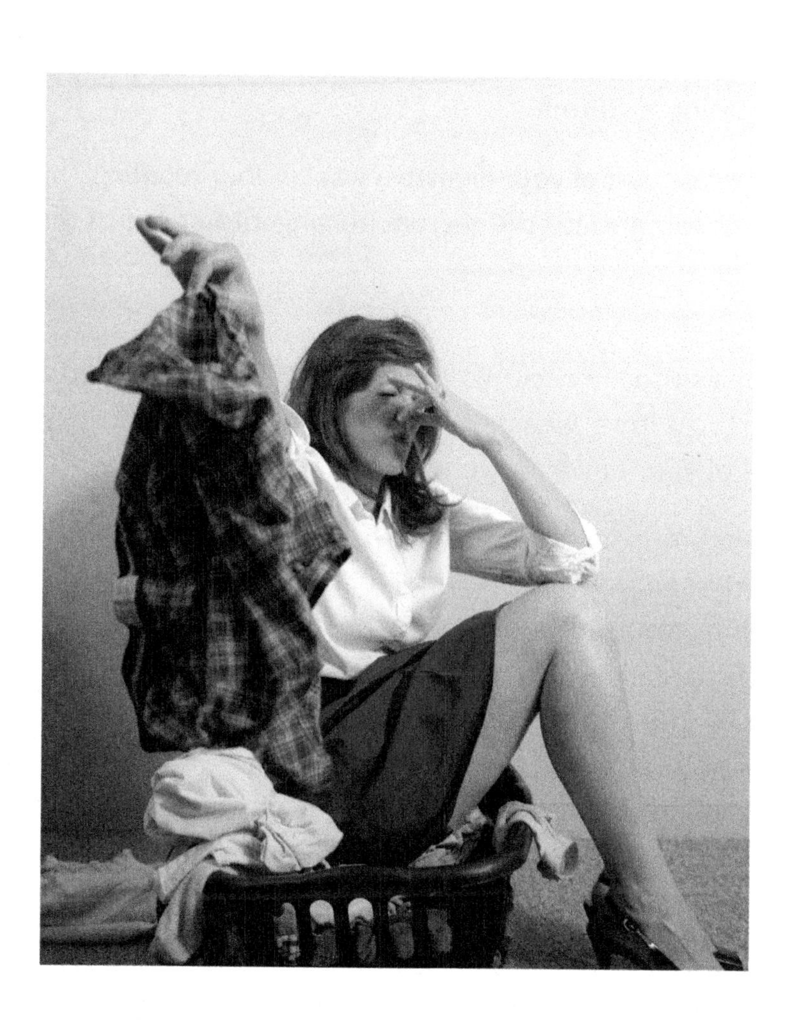

Stinky Problem

Oh dear! What could be more embarrassing than to poop your pants?

It's embarrassing to poop your pants!

Nature devised a nifty disposal system to eliminate solid waste from your body. As you generate fecal material, it passes through your large intestine into the lower part called your rectum. There it accumulates. But this waste should be held in place until, intermittently, the tightly held muscle of your anus relaxes and you have a bowel movement to empty it out.

> **Coming to Terms**
>
> The last part of your digestive tract is your ***rectum***. The medical term for the rectum bulging into or out of the vaginal wall is ***rectocele***.

Rectoceles usually occur as a result of injuries sustained during childbirth. With a weakened or bulging rectum, you may lose control of your bowel movements.

Your rectum is located next to your vaginal cavity. When the wall between your vagina and rectum becomes too weak to hold your lower bowel in place, the bowel protrudes out of its normal channel and bulges into your vagina. Sometimes it even bulges all the way out of your vagina. A large bulge into the vaginal wall can cause so much pressure that your rectal muscle gets fatigued and can't hold back the storm of fecal material from your bowel. Then, fecal material flows right out into your undies.

Again, Just the Opposite

If it's not one thing, it's another. What if you're constantly constipated?

Granny Vagina Dilemma: "I can't poop at all."

SYMPTOM: A bulging bowel can become an obstructed bowel, making bowel movements a nightmare.

Major Gridlock

A leaky rectum is bad, but sometimes just the opposite happens. When your pelvic floor muscles and connective tissue become too weak, your rectum can protrude into your vagina, creating an obstruction and making it difficult for fecal material to pass. It's as if the stool takes a detour through the vaginal hernia before going out in the right direction. When this obstruction occurs, you will find it hard to initiate a bowel movement, especially if you are constipated.

Some women must reach into their vagina with their finger and push the bulge down and away from the vaginal opening in order to have a bowel movement.

Blame the Baby?

Pelvic organ prolapse results from injury to the muscles or supporting tissue of the pelvic floor. The main cause of this type of injury is childbearing. Researchers estimate that approximately one-half of all the women who have had a baby will develop some degree of muscle and tissue damage, eventually leading to pelvic organ prolapse.

The main cause of pelvic muscle injury is childbearing.

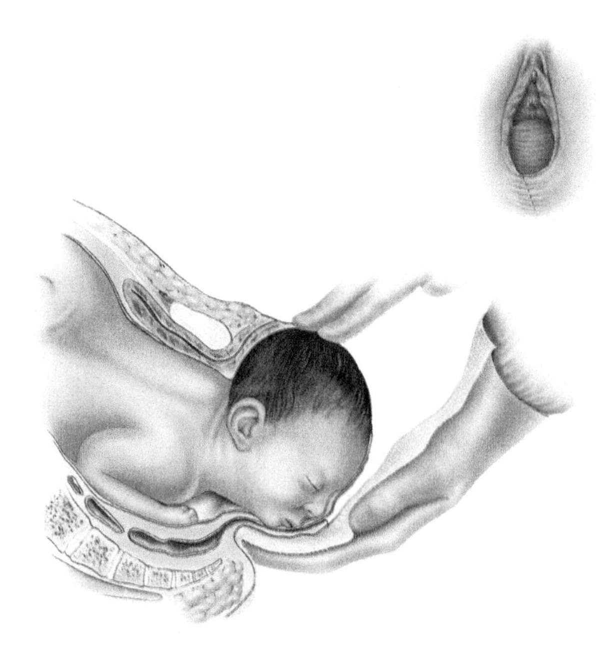

Women who have had a Cesarean delivery have less risk for pelvic support problems than those women who have had one or more vaginal deliveries. During childbirth, as the baby passes through the birth canal, the muscles, tissue, and ligaments stretch, pull apart, and separate and may become weakened. This weakening gradually worsens, and in later years, may allow the pelvic organs to drop from their normal positions.

"But I've never had children."

Occasionally, this weakening of the muscles and tissue occurs in women who have never had children. In these women, pelvic support problems may be attributable to unusual strain placed on the supporting tissue by such things as difficult bowel movements, chronic coughing or intense physical activity.

Strains on Supporting Tissue

- Vaginal delivery
- Difficult bowel movements

- Chronic coughing
- Intense physical activity
- Heredity (inherited weakness of the supporting tissue)
- Prior pelvic surgery
- Aging, menopause
- Obesity, being overweight

Granny Vagina Dilemma: "Something's pressuring my pelvis."

SYMPTOMS: If the top of your vagina gives way just a little, your only symptom might be a little pressure. If the top should sag extremely low, however, you will be able to see it sticking out of your vagina.

Your Roof's Caving In

Your vagina is a tube-like structure surrounded by muscles. When those muscles weaken and lose their support, the top of the tube (the ***apex***) can come bulging down into the lower vagina (like a roof caving in). This condition is ***vaginal vault prolapse***. You may experience pelvic pressure that gets worse as the day goes on. Or it may be brought on with standing, lifting or coughing.

Inside Out

Vaginal vault prolapse occurs most often in women who have had their uterus removed (hysterectomy). After a hysterectomy, the normal support from the uterus is no longer in place, and the vagina can simply turn inside out.

The degree of vaginal vault prolapse varies: the top of your vagina may fall just a little, or it may cave in a great deal. It may sag so low that it bulges all the way outside your vaginal opening. Severe forms of this condition lead to more severe problems.

And That Prolapse Can Lead to ...

SYMPTOMS: Sensing pressure as everything in your pelvic cavity gets squeezed out of place, and possible digestive problems.

Not a Small Problem

Not only is vaginal vault prolapse a problem in itself, but also the expanding space, which results when the top of your vagina falls, is an invitation for surrounding organs to push into that space. (Nature abhors a vacuum.) Bladder and bowel function may be affected.

Nature abhors a vacuum.

When vaginal vault prolapse allows your small intestine to push down into the expanding space, it creates an ***enterocele***, a bulge pushing against the back wall of your vagina. Bulging can occur from the front, back or top.

Coming to Terms

Small intestine prolapse is an ***enterocele***.

Progression of Symptoms

Symptoms of pelvic support problems leading to prolapse can be elusive at first. As muscles and tissue around your pelvic organs begin to stretch and weaken, you might experience only minor symptoms or no visible symptoms at all. You may be surprised when I tell you things have begun to give way down there.

One of the first signs of prolapse you may encounter is a bulge of tissue inside your vagina. If the bulge of tissue is visible, it is often red and sore and can be alarming. You may experience vaginal discharge, spotting or bleeding.

You might find it becomes more difficult to insert a tampon. And inserting a penis? Well, if you have a male sex partner, that's often the most embarrassing symptom to admit. All sex becomes difficult when there is a bulge in the way.

How sexy can you feel when sex is painful?

As muscles and tissue stretch and give way even more, this weakness causes a sensation of pelvic heaviness or fullness. The pelvic pressure often gets worse as the day goes on.

Your symptoms will become more severe when your inner organs begin to drop. Lower back pain intensifies. Women describe it as a pulling or aching, or pressure in the lower abdomen or pelvis.

Gradually, symptoms become more specific, depending on which organ is affected.

The Good News and the Bad News

How About the Bad News First?

HERE'S THE BAD NEWS: Many women suffer unnecessarily. All too often, the Granny Vagina Dilemmas we've been discussing in this chapter go undetected by healthcare workers who aren't examining you closely enough.

Many women suffer unnecessarily.

Or, worse yet, obvious cases of pelvic organ prolapse are actually misdiagnosed.

Case in Point

I treated a lady who was referred to me by her trainer at the gym. Every time she jumped, she peed. Tragically, she had suffered this problem for years, thinking it was just something she had to live with.

Another doctor had assured this patient that everything was fine, when it wasn't. Her symptoms of bladder prolapse were brushed off as "overflow incontinence—you just don't empty your bladder well."

She had been prescribed ***tibial nerve stimulation***, a treatment that helps with the constant sensation of urgency (which she didn't have). Of course, this treatment did not provide a remedy for her embarrassing problem: her bladder was falling down into her vagina, causing her to lose a squirt of urine every time she jumped. This type of damage often requires repair with surgery to the weakened muscles and tissue, securing the bladder back up in its proper place. The standard of care is a ***sling procedure*** (a piece of material surgically implanted under the urethra to support it).

Coming to Terms

Sling procedure—Procedure in which a piece of material is surgically implanted under the urethra to support it.

And Now the Good News

THE GOOD NEWS is that appropriate diagnosis and treatment will often restore you to a life free of the aggravation and discomfort associated with Granny Vagina Dilemmas.

Appropriate Diagnosis

Diagnosis of your Granny Vagina Dilemmas includes taking a thorough history of your health over the years. You'll also undergo a physical examination, as well as other tests, depending on the circumstances.

Coming Up Next: Definitive Treatment

It's time to take your Granny Vagina Dilemmas along to the next section: "Part Two: Now What Happens?" where you will learn about treatment options for prolapse.

For milder cases, when your organs are not yet too far displaced, there are a variety of non-surgical treatments that may provide relief. For advanced cases of pelvic organ prolapse, however, the definitive treatment may be surgical correction of specific defects.

Part

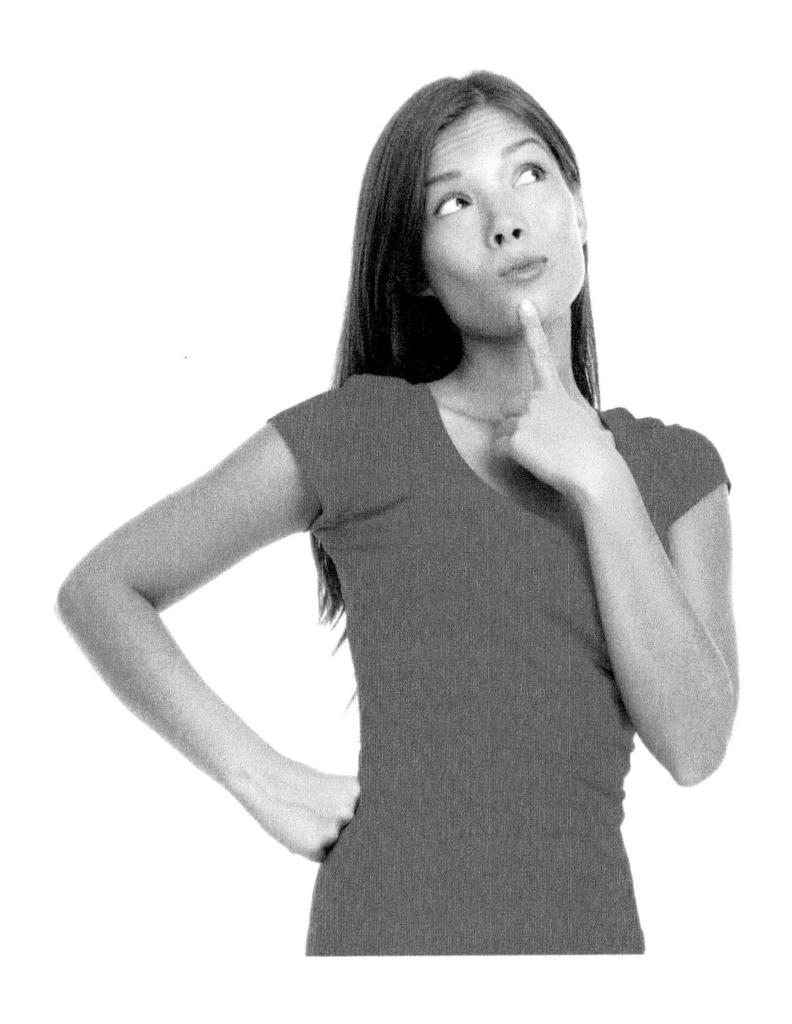

Two

Now What Happens?

Chapter Four

What's a Woman to Do?

Granny Vagina Dilemma: "Now what happens?"

While I was putting together that last chapter on all those prolapses, I gave my sister a copy to proofread. She sent it back with the comment, "Oh Great! We've learned all about Granny Vaginas. What if you think you have one? Now what happens?"

My answer to all of you who raise that question: why merely cope with your Granny Vagina Dilemma? Work with your doctor to diagnose what's wrong; then fix it. Develop a treatment plan that will improve your quality of life—you're worth it.

Work with your doctor to diagnose what's wrong; then fix it.

First Things First: Diagnosis

The key to your treatment plan starts with diagnosis; we have to find the exact cause of your problem. If you're due for your annual exam, schedule it. If you're not yet due for your annual exam, call your doctor's office and ask for an appointment for a pelvic problem.

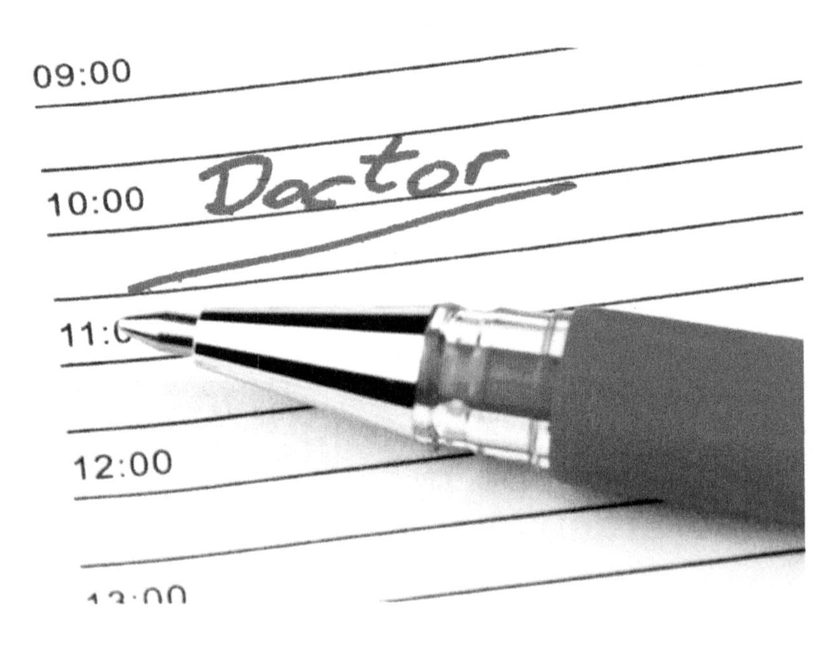

Work with Your Doctor

If you're a patient in my office, you'll be given a thorough examination. I've provided an overview of the annual exam basics you can expect in chapter fourteen, "Your Annual Wellness/ Pelvic Screening Examination." Because vaginal problems are my specialty, I focus on Granny Vaginas with every patient who comes to see me.

In your community, shop around for a healthcare provider who knows which symptoms to look for and how to decipher signs of Granny Vagina Dilemmas. Many gynecological surgeons have extensive training in this area, and they take the time to do excellent pelvic examinations. How fortunate for you and your vagina if you have access to such a knowledgeable person!

Shop around for a knowledgeable healthcare provider.

Unfortunately, that's not always the case. If you find you must work with someone you suspect may not be genuinely knowledgeable about vaginas—or who seems to be focusing on something else and not your possible problems—don't despair. You can steer them in the right direction.

Do Your Homework—Be Prepared

When you go for your exam, be prepared to bring up all your concerns. Describe your symptoms specifically. Ask questions and don't be satisfied until you have confidence in the answers you receive. Feel free to confide whatever is on your mind. Medical professionals who work in this area usually take pride in their field of expertise and should appreciate it when you are completely open with them.

Treatment Options

Granny Vagina Dilemma: "Am I headed for surgery?"

Your condition could require surgery; or when symptoms are first detected, we might be able to treat your prolapse with something more conservative. To help us decide, we'll look at several factors:

How Bad Off Are You?

What's the extent of your prolapse? If your condition is severe, more aggressive treatment may be necessary.

Are You Healthy?

How's your general health? Are you vigorous for your age, or frail?

Sexually Active?

And what about sex—are you (or do you look forward to being) sexually active?

Looking into Your Future

Do you want to have children in the future? If so, you might consider holding off on surgery until after you give birth to your children. Discuss pregnancy and pelvic support problems with your doctor.

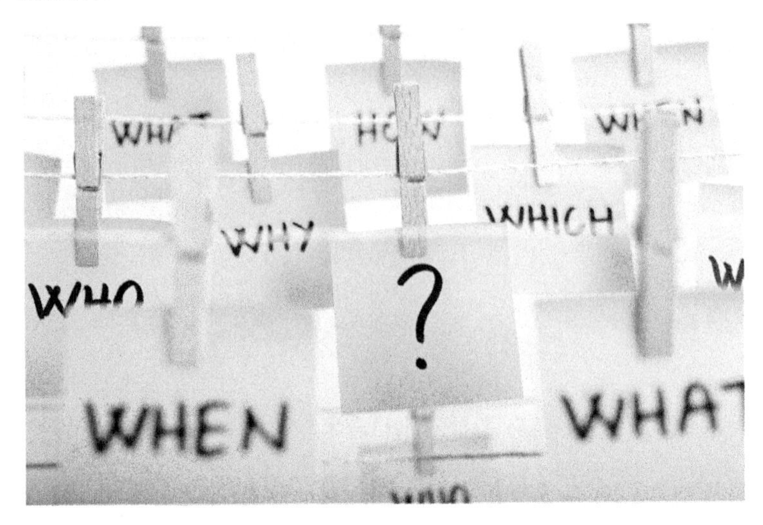

Granny Vagina Dilemma: "How many treatment options do I have?"

The short answer: a whole bunch. No one treatment will be right for all women. Let's start by describing easier, nonsurgical treatments (appropriate if your Granny Vagina symptoms are slight).

Nonsurgical Treatments when Symptoms Are Slight

Maybe Just Symptom Management for Now

We may find your vaginal problem is not severe enough to need immediate treatment. In that case, I will keep track of your problem at regular check-ups, and treatment can be started at a later time if symptoms become bothersome.

Relief of Specific Symptoms

Relieving specific symptoms may be as simple as making changes in your diet and lifestyle.

Relief of symptoms may be simple.

Incontinence

Mild cases of embarrassing incontinence may be lessened by limiting your fluid intake, especially those drinks that contain caffeine. Sometimes it's helpful to empty your bladder at scheduled times to "train" it to wait.

Bowel Issues

Preventing constipation and avoiding excessive straining during bowel movements are especially important. When increasing the amount of fiber in your diet isn't effective, I may prescribe a laxative or other medication that softens stools.

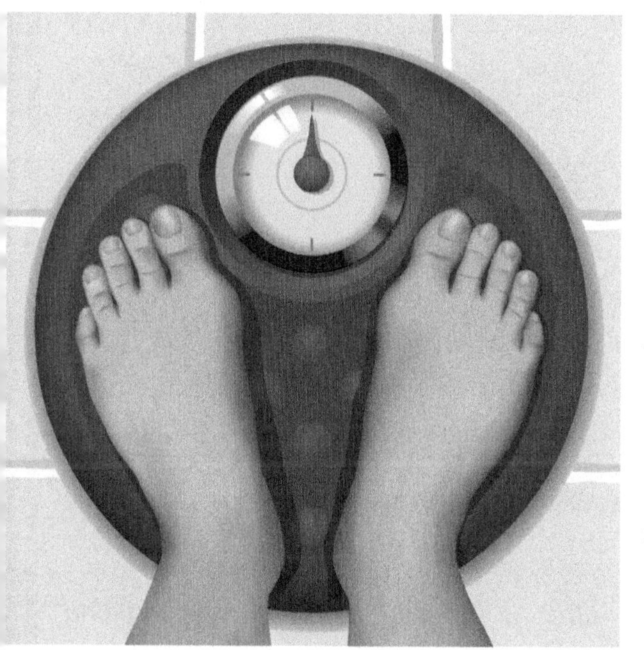

Excess Weight

Your prolapse symptoms may be aggravated if you are overweight or obese. In addition to improving your overall health, losing weight might help relieve those symptoms.

Special Exercises Might Do the Trick

If your vaginal tissue is otherwise healthy, exercises for toning the pelvic floor might be helpful. These exercises specifically aim at strengthening muscles inside the vagina, those muscles surrounding the opening of your vagina, and those muscles surrounding your urethra and rectum. In mild cases of prolapse, exercise might be the only treatment needed. A special set of exercises developed by Dr. Kegel (and called, appropriately enough, ***Kegels***) are regularly prescribed.

Coming to Terms

Kegels are a set of exercises for strengthening otherwise healthy vaginal muscles.

To be effective, Kegels need to be done daily. It usually takes a period of four to six weeks to notice any improvement.

How to Do Kegels

Concentrate on the muscles you use to stop the flow of urine; squeeze them tight, pulling your vagina and rectum up and back.

Hold on to your squeeze for up to ten seconds, then release and relax.

Do fifty of these contractions per day. It may be troublesome to do fifty Kegels all at once; I usually recommend doing ten Kegel contractions at a time. When driving, you could get in the habit of doing ten at every stop sign or traffic signal.

Be mindful not to squeeze other muscles: stomach, thigh, or buttocks.

Breathe normally when doing your Kegels; avoid holding your breath.

Enhance Those Kegels

Weighted vaginal cones can be ordered to enhance the effectiveness of Kegel exercises. They come in sets with incrementally increasing weights to place inside the cone. Think of lifting weights at the gym: you progress to heavier weights as your muscles become stronger. The same principle applies to the weighted vaginal cones. Sort of like Super Kegels!

Be patient. Significant improvement often takes at least six weeks of daily use. You should use weighted cones indefinitely to maintain results.

Not for Injuries

Note that Kegel exercises are for strengthening healthy muscles. They can't repair significant injuries to your vaginal muscles and tissue. More about this Dilemma in chapter six, "Yo Thang Be Raggedy."

Referral for Pelvic Floor Therapy

Sometimes it's appropriate to recommend working with a physical therapist who has special training in techniques to strengthen the pelvic muscles. The most common techniques include:

Biofeedback

Biofeedback involves placing a device into your vagina or rectum along with electrodes stuck to your ***perineal area*** (the surface region between your vagina and your anus). Feedback (using lights or sound) helps you identify when you are contracting the proper muscles needed to strengthen the pelvic floor.

Electrical Stimulation

This device uses a gentle electrical current to cause your pelvic floor muscles to contract.

Hold That Prolapse In with a Pessary Device

Pessaries are devices placed inside your vagina to mechanically push up or hold up prolapsing tissue. Pessaries come in all shapes and sizes. You and I will need to assess your Granny Vagina Dilemma, choose the proper pessary for your particular problem, and fit one to your size.

Don't Do This

In olden days, women often resorted to using things they had on hand to place inside their vagina and hold the prolapse up. Potatoes were a common everyday item used for this purpose. I certainly don't advocate this home-grown remedy as an option.

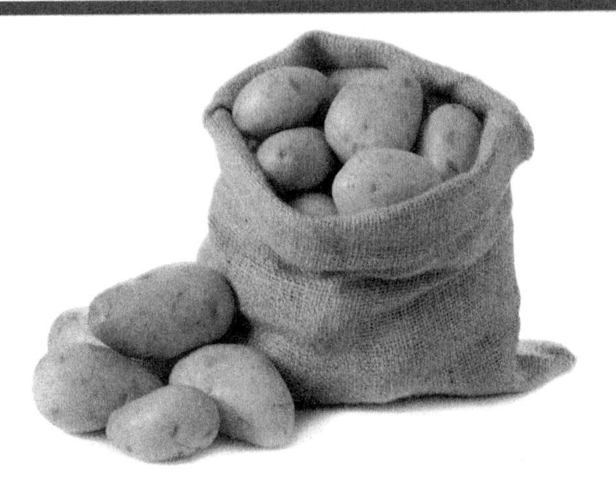

In today's medical practice, pessaries are generally reserved for use in specific situations. Some examples are:

- For elderly women who are too frail or infirm to withstand a surgical repair

- As a temporizing measure to get someone through until definitive treatment can be performed; examples might be a woman who is pregnant, or for use during treatment of thin, pale, or weak vaginal tissue with estrogen
- As an option for women who do not wish to have surgical repairs

Note that some women won't be pessary candidates if their vaginal opening is too large or prolapse too severe. The pessary could simply fall out, or be pushed out, once she stands up.

Estrogen Therapy (ERT)

Sometimes, restoring adequate estrogen to vaginal and vulvar tissue is all that's needed to treat mild cases of Granny Vagina. I am limiting this description of estrogen to our discussion of non-surgical treatments for Granny Vagina Dilemmas typically found in women before menopause. You'll find a more in-depth commentary in chapter eleven, "Hormone Basics."

Estrogen Is Really, Really Important

Vaginal Tissue and Hormones

Inspection of your vaginal tissue can act as a window into the hormone health of your entire body.

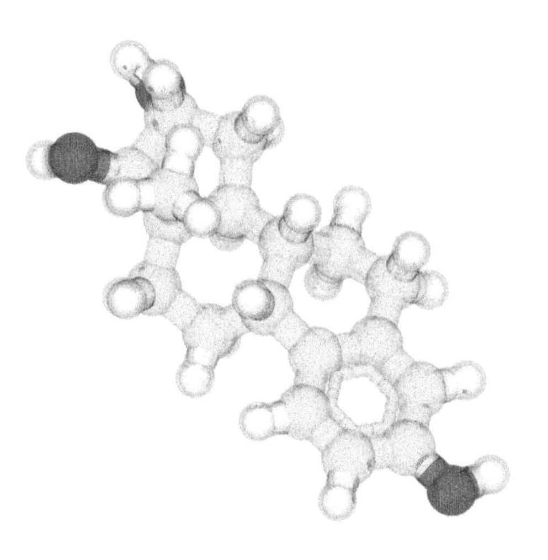

The tissue of your vagina exquisitely depends on adequate levels of the hormone estrogen to maintain thickness, elasticity, moisture, and strength. Estrogen is also essential for ***pH balance*** (a measure of the acid or base quality) and for infection control.

Forms of Estrogen

Estrogen*—a woman's defining natural female sex hormone. It is responsible for ovulation, menstrual periods and pregnancy. Estrogen also influences essential body functions. Estrogen is produced in a woman's body in several forms:*

> ***(E_1) Estrone****—the dominant form of estrogen in women after menopause, and in men.*
> ***(E_2) Estradiol****—a form of hormone present in the ovaries and the dominant estrogen in the body prior to menopause.*
> ***(E_3) Estriol****—the estrogen produced during pregnancy.*

Progesterone*—the natural female sex hormone that acts within the womb and placenta in connection with pregnancy.*

Choosing Your Estrogen

Many factors will be taken into consideration when deciding whether you should use estrogen therapy for your Granny Vagina Dilemma, and what form would be most appropriate for your individual situation. Estrogen can be supplemented either systemically (throughout your entire body) or locally (just in your vagina).

Locally Applied Estrogen Options Available from a Commercial Pharmacy

Here is a sampling of estrogen replacements that are available today from your local pharmacy with a prescription; undoubtedly, more will become available as pharmaceutical manufacturers introduce new products.

Note

This book offers general information and is not intended to be an exhaustive discourse on estrogen use. Each pharmaceutical company provides inserts with its estrogen products, which disclose in detail important safety information and intended uses. You should read this information before beginning estrogen therapy.

Vaginal Tablets

Vagifem® tablets are small bioidentical estradiol pills that are positioned high in the vagina with an applicator. Typical dosing would be one tablet nightly for two weeks, then two to three times per week thereafter.

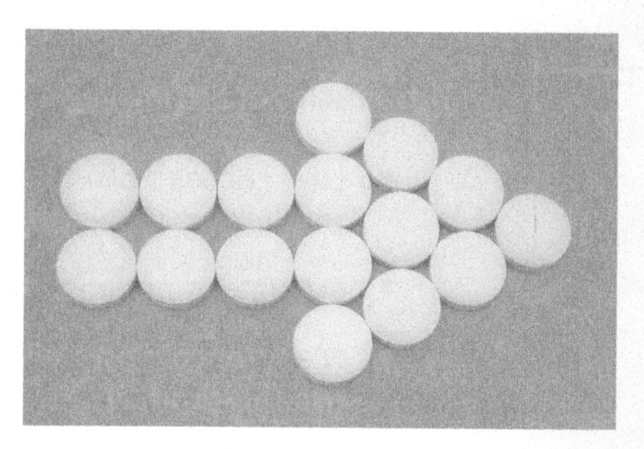

Coming to Terms

Bioidentical means the hormones have a molecular structure identical to your body's own natural female sex hormones.

Advantages of Vagifem:

- Vagifem tablets provide small estrogen doses that do not get absorbed throughout the rest of the body.
- Many oncologists allow breast cancer patients to use this form of local vaginal estrogen therapy.
- This estrogen does not cause the lining of the uterus to grow.

Disadvantages of Vagifem:

- Tablets must be inserted regularly.
- Sometimes the vagina is too dry for tablets to dissolve.
- This product is not generic; price may be a concern.

Vaginal Rings

Estring® vaginal ring is a flexible ring impregnated with bioidentical estradiol. The device remains in the vagina for up to three months at a time (inserted much like a diaphragm contraceptive device).

Advantages of Estring vaginal ring:

- Low doses of estrogen are continuously released throughout the entire three-month period.
- Estrogen is not absorbed systemically.
- Many oncologists allow their breast cancer patients to use this product.
- This estrogen does not cause the lining of the uterus to grow.

Disadvantages of Estring vaginal ring:

- Ring may fall out if the vaginal opening is too wide or the prolapse too severe.
- Ring might be too large to fit comfortably in some women.
- This product is not generic; price may be a concern.

Femring® vaginal ring is a bioidentical estrogen ring applied vaginally for up to three months at a time. It should be noted that Femring comes in doses appropriate for systemic absorption (going throughout the body).

Vaginal Creams

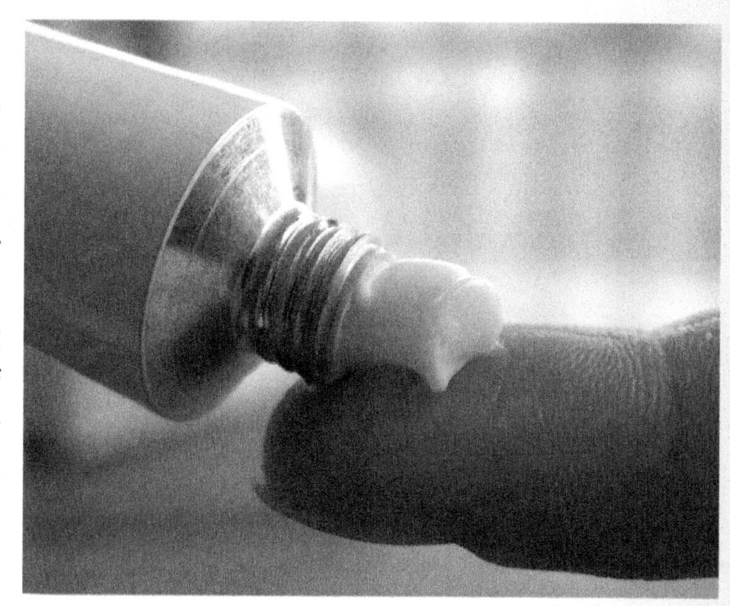

Estrace® vaginal cream is a bioidentical estradiol cream that can be applied to external genitalia or applied vaginally with an applicator. Typical dosing is one to four grams of cream, applied daily for two weeks, then two to three times per week thereafter.

Advantages of Estrace vaginal cream:

- Cream is often soothing.
- This product will be absorbed even on dry tissue.

Disadvantages of Estrace vaginal cream:

- Cream is messy.
- It must be applied often.
- It has the potential for more systemic absorption and might not be appropriate for women with a history of breast or uterine cancers.
- Use of Estrace vaginal cream may require monitoring the thickness of the uterus lining or the addition of progesterone therapy.
- This product is not generic; price may be a concern.

Premarin® vaginal cream is a conjugated estrogen cream (meaning it is a union of compounds). Patients apply the cream vaginally or to external genitalia and they typically use it daily for two weeks, then one to two times per week thereafter.

> **Coming to Terms**
>
> ***Conjugated*** means formed by a union of compounds.

Advantages of Premarin vaginal cream:

- Cream is often soothing.
- This product will be absorbed even on dry tissue.

Disadvantages of Premarin vaginal cream:

- This product is not bioidentical. Its estrogen originates in the urine of pregnant horses.
- Cream is messy.
- It must be applied often.
- It has the potential for more systemic absorption and might not be appropriate for women with a history of breast or uterine cancers.
- Use of Premarin vaginal cream may require monitoring the thickness of the uterus lining or the addition of progesterone therapy.
- This product is not generic; price may be a concern.

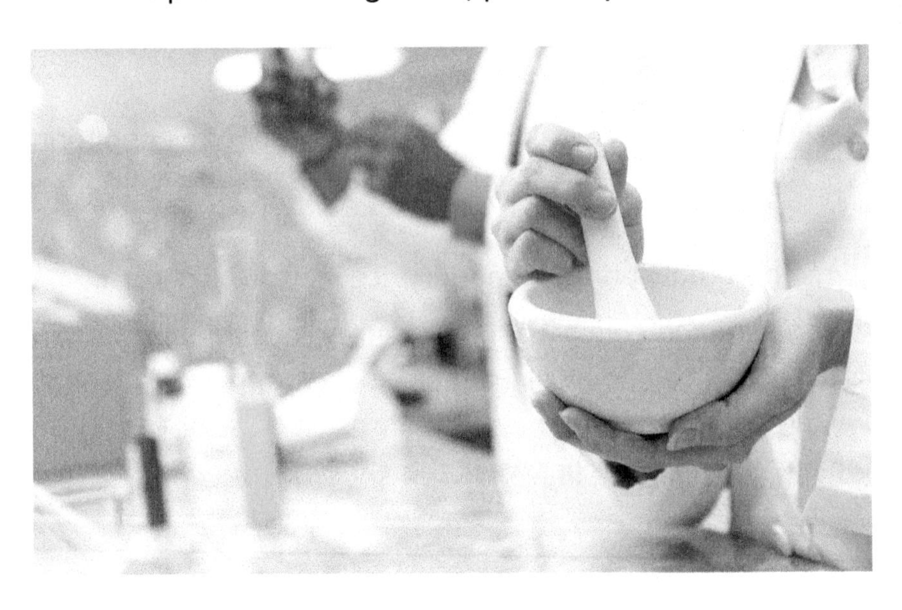

Locally Applied Estrogen Options Available Only from a Compounding Pharmacy

Compounding pharmacies are specialty pharmacies that make custom preparations based on formulas prescribed by physicians.

Compounding pharmacies make custom preparations.

Some advantages of compounding pharmacies:

- Compounding pharmacies can provide drugs or hormones not manufactured commercially.
- They can provide hormones and individualized drugs in combinations that are not commercially available at traditional pharmacies.
- Often used when commercial preparations are not suitable: for example, when a patient needs non-standard doses or different routes of delivery.

Some disadvantages of compounding pharmacies:

- There is more room for error in making up each "recipe."
- Insurance might not cover the cost.

E_3 vaginal cream or suppositories

E_3 is the type of estrogen known as estriol. The vagina, vulva, and urethra are all rich with E_3 receptors and respond well to local treatment. E_3 cream or suppositories are available only from a compounding pharmacy.

And if Nonsurgical Options Don't Work ...

In the next chapter, "Surgery from a Patient's Point of View," we'll move along to surgical treatments for more drastic Dilemmas, ending with what's liable to happen if you let your condition progress to that worst Granny Vagina Disaster—prolapsed uterus. (Hint: how would you like to have your vagina put out of commission forever?)

Chapter Five

Surgery from a Patient's Point of View

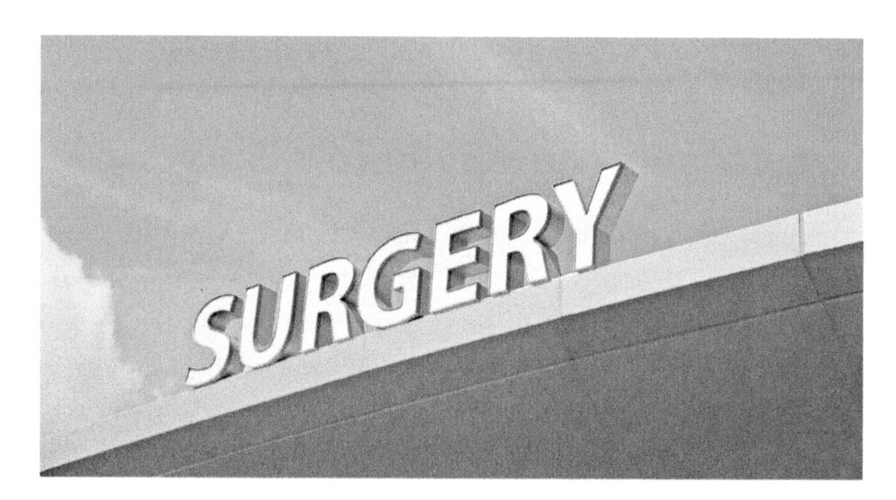

Restoring You to Normal Health

You and I want your lady-parts to be restored to normal health. And we want them to stay that way, functioning the way nature intended. After we've explored your nonsurgical options, if we find your Granny Vagina Dilemma can't be brought under control by nonsurgical means, then you're a candidate for surgical correction. Don't panic. Although all surgery should be taken seriously, pelvic repair surgery is common.

Pelvic repair is a common surgery.

Make an Election

Most pelvic repairs are completed with elective surgery—not urgent or done in response to an emergency (except in rare cases).

This election doesn't imply that your surgery is not medically indicated, just that you can choose the timing for your surgery. You can elect to have it when it suits you and your schedule.

Knowledge Is Power

I've titled this chapter "Surgery from a Patient's Point of View" because I find this information is what my patients are concerned about: "What's this surgery going to mean for me, Dr. King?" Speaking for myself, I always feel less anxious about an upcoming event when I know ahead of time just what to expect. With that thought in mind, let's take you on a tour of your surgery experience, from start to finish.

Estrogen Therapy before Surgery

The goal for both of us is to make this repair last a lifetime, so that you won't have to come back again and again. This repair requires healthy tissue, before and after surgery, for the stitches to hold. If your vaginal tissue is in good condition, then we're ready to go.

But if your vaginal tissue is too thin, any attempt at stitching it together would be like trying to sew tissue paper to tissue paper. That's why, at times, estrogen therapy is the essential first step before surgical repair can even be considered.

Stitching too thin vaginal tissue is like sewing tissue paper to tissue paper.

This Therapy Might Take a While

If your vaginal tissue lacks estrogen and becomes thin, pale, and weak, you're simply not yet ready for surgical treatment. Once you begin estrogen therapy to correct this condition, it might take as long as six to eight weeks before the treatment restores your tissue health to pre-surgical requirements. (Your vagina didn't lose its estrogen overnight, and it takes time to restore and heal its tissue.) Be patient, and remember—our goal is a lifetime repair.

Prepare for Success

To ensure your best chances for a smooth and successful surgery, there are things you can do to prepare yourself.

I strive to set my patients up for success.

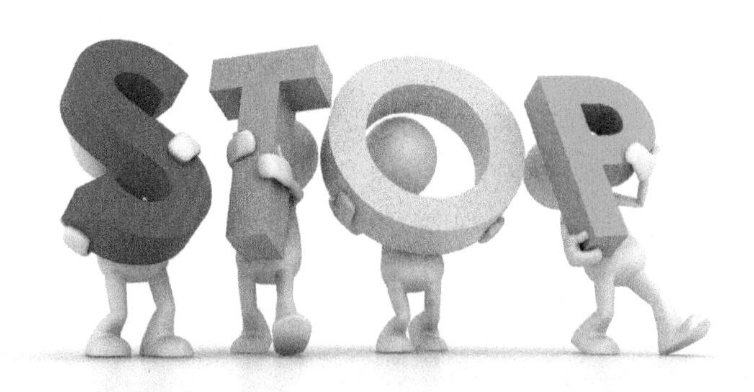

Stop That

You must discontinue using supplements that act as blood thinners and could cause excessive bruising, bleeding, or other complications. This list includes Aspirin (and any formulas containing Aspirin), Ibuprofen, Vitamin E, and so forth.

If you are a smoker, you must stop smoking at least two weeks before and after surgery. Nicotine can impair healing and circulation, and smoking decreases the amount of oxygen your tissue receives.

Restrict alcohol intake. Don't drink alcohol in excess for several weeks before and after surgery.

Be as Healthy as You Can Be

Stay hydrated by drinking lots of water in the days leading up to your surgery. Arrive for surgery well

Arrive well rested and well nourished.

rested and well nourished. (But do not eat or drink anything after midnight the night prior to surgery, unless expressly instructed to do so.)

If you have any pressing medical conditions—such as asthma, and so forth—they should be under tight control.

Are Your Bowels Ready?

When it comes to pelvic surgery, you should also pay particular attention to your bowels. Do not come into your surgery constipated, as it will only get worse afterwards and may compromise your repair. I recommend that you start a stool softener several days ahead of time. Increasing fiber in your diet also helps.

The Best Laid Plans

Before surgery day, catch up on grocery shopping, laundry, house cleaning, and any extra projects from your job. Fill your pain prescriptions and place them within easy reach of where you will be resting.

Make sure you will have adequate help at home, especially for activities that would require lifting. And if you have young children, find someone to assist with their care.

Arrange for someone to take you home from your surgery and be with you for at least the first day. Then make plans to take it easy for up to several weeks to allow your body the time and energy to heal properly.

Consult and Give Consent

You and I will meet for a pre-surgery consultation in my office where we will go over all the particulars of your upcoming surgery. We'll review your medical records and note whether all necessary tests are in order.

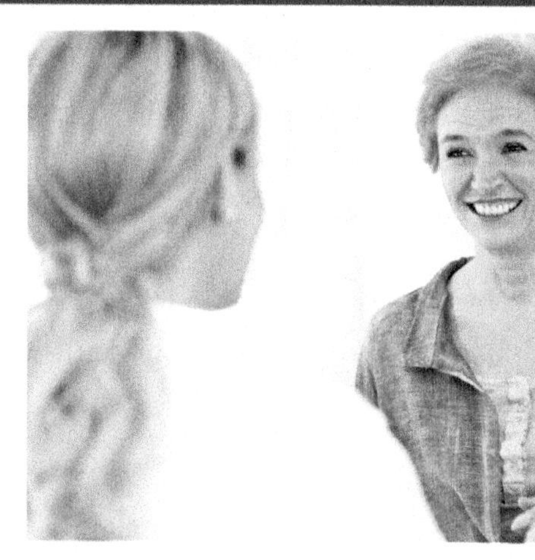

Now is the time for you to be open; share your concerns and any information that may pertain to your health. You should tell me anything I don't already know about your medical history, and all the medications, vitamins, and herbs you are taking. Even if you don't think they're important, some substances can affect blood clotting or other important functions. We'll go over the medications and herbal supplements that you must avoid prior to your procedure.

Important objectives of our consultation are to be certain you know what your condition is, what surgery is scheduled, and why. You should understand the expected outcome and be aware of the risks involved with your particular surgery. We'll discuss specific details, such as the type of anesthesia you'll be given. And I'll inform you about restrictions you'll need to observe once you return home: for example, lifting, bathing, and resuming activity with your sexual partner.

Pain management is important, and you'll want to follow instructions on how to progress through your recovery with a minimum of discomfort. I'll give you your post-op pain prescriptions the day prior to surgery so that you can fill them ahead of time and have them ready when you need them at home.

With everything in order, you must give informed consent in writing for surgery to be done, and we'll be ready for the big day.

Day of Surgery

If you have an early morning slot on the surgery schedule, I would advise having everything in order at home the night before. Choose to wear loose, comfortable clothing (something easy to get into when it's time to go home).

You'll arrive one and a half hours before your scheduled surgery time. Stop at Outpatient Registration and register with the hospital, then go to Day Surgery. From here on, all you have to do is smile and relax while lots of efficient staff persons take over and lead you through your pre-op.

From here on, all you have to do is smile and relax.

I will come in to talk with you one more time and ask if you have any questions. The anesthesiologist will pay you a visit.

After the nurse starts your injection (IV) with a saline solution, you'll be wheeled into the operating room. Then it's onto the operating table, where you'll be hooked up to monitors for vital functions such as heart rate and blood pressure.

Here's the pleasant part: medicine will be introduced into your IV, and you'll drift off to sleep.

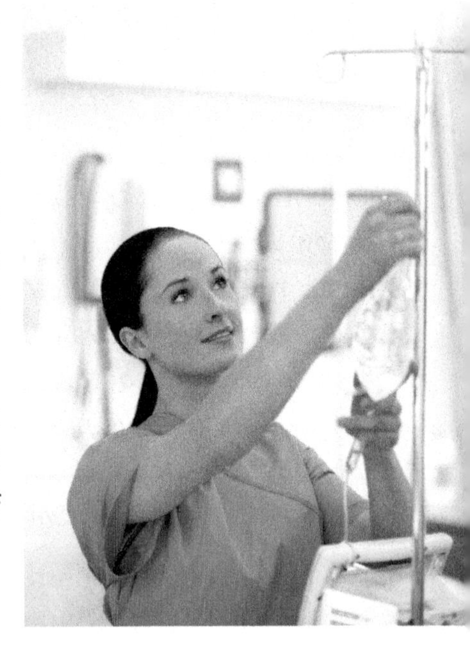

A Brief Description of Your Surgery

I'm not going to go into technical jargon and detail about what actually takes place during your surgical procedure. After all, you'll be asleep and blissfully unaware the whole time, anyway.

But I want my patients to be informed about some of the more significant aspects.

Surgery: Easy to Disaster

Don't put off Granny Vagina Dilemma until disaster strikes.

I can't stress enough the importance of choosing to have your Granny Vagina Dilemma taken care of before it gets out of hand and not putting it off until disaster strikes.

For example, think about going to the dentist. Do you have a cavity? Deal with it now with a small filling and it's no big deal. Ignore it until tooth disaster strikes—wait until pain and infection set in—then you may need a difficult root canal.

It's much the same when it comes to surgical treatment options for pelvic organ disorders: you're faced with a continuum of difficulty, which only gets more difficult the longer you wait.

Easier Surgery for Granny Vagina Dilemmas

Nip and Tuck and Tighten

We'll start with the easier scenario: you've come to see me when you have a pelvic organ bulging out of place into your vagina, but it isn't hanging all the way out. When your prolapse is bad enough to fix, but not yet Disaster stage, the surgical treatment is straightforward—mostly nip and tuck and tighten. Basically, here's how your surgery will go:

Once you're sleeping soundly, I'll introduce a ***pudendal*** nerve block (on one of your pelvic nerves) with long-acting local anesthetic, which will keep you comfortable for the first eighteen to twenty-four hours after surgery. Then I'll inject tumescent solution (saline, lidocane and epinephrine) into the vaginal tissue to decrease bleeding and make tissue dissection easier.

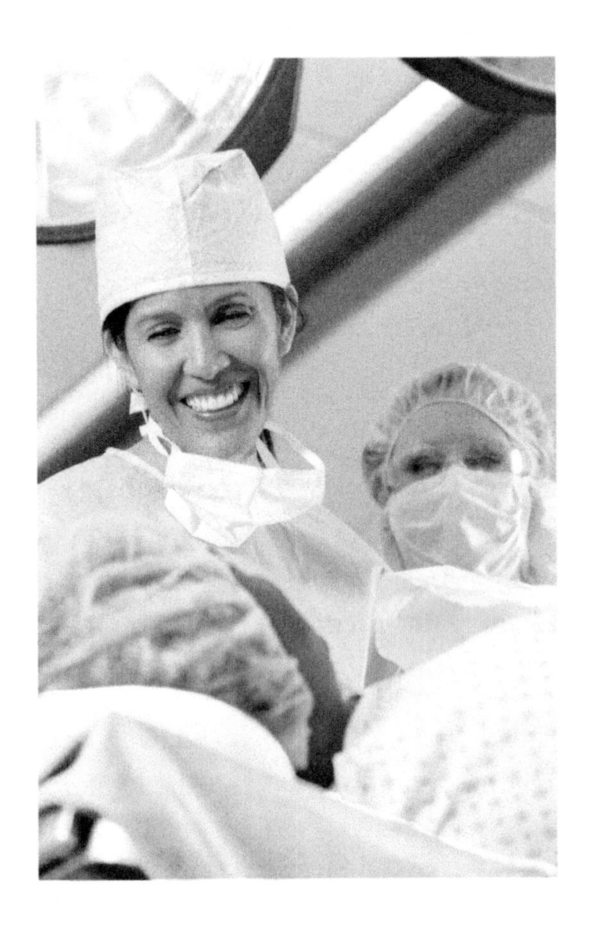

A Word about Surgical Techniques

Traditional: *During graduate medical training, gynecology students are taught surgical methods of vaginal repair that are often quite invasive. This conventional surgery may cause patients to suffer long and painful recovery. I prefer not to use such methods.*

Laser Surgery: *I have completed specialized training in a new method of laser surgery. Where appropriate, I employ a laser as my surgical instrument. The laser provides precise, controlled accuracy and affords a relatively bloodless technique.*

Your bulging organ will be re-situated back to its proper position, then stitched in place. Any excess vaginal tissue will be removed and the skin layer closed.

In completion, I'll institute a procedure I developed (***Vaginal Regenalift™***), injecting your own platelet-rich-plasma along all inside and outside incision lines to promote rapid healing. This healing allows you to resume your daily activities in a short period of time.

That Pee-Pee Problem

In chapter three we talked about stress urinary incontinence (when you're unable to control bursts of urine with sudden stress on your bladder). Currently, the "gold standard" treatment is a sling procedure, placing an approved type of sling under your urethra to support it.

If you're only having a sling procedure, you may be released to go home the same day. Other pelvic prolapse repairs often require an overnight stay in the hospital.

Surgical Repair of Granny Vagina Disaster: Procidentia

Obviously, once your connective tissue gives way—lets loose, pops its coil—I can't simply do a nip or tuck and expect everything to stay in its proper place. Something has to be done to tie or tack your prolapsing organ back where it belongs. If you wait

Coming to Terms

Procidentia is a medical term with a meaning similar to prolapse: the complete falling down of an organ from its normal anatomical position.

until your insides fall out, I have no choice but to resort to measures that may include some sort of mesh, and permanent sutures connected to stronger structures than those tissues that gave way.

A Word about Pelvic Mesh

Surgeons commonly use mesh when native tissue fails; for instance, in hernia operations they often insert mesh to reinforce the hernia area. Pelvic mesh products were developed to augment pelvic organ prolapse repair. I try to avoid using mesh products during my repairs unless faced with dreaded Granny Vagina Disasters like procidentia. In these cases, catastrophic connective tissue failure requires drastic corrective measures. You might have seen those ads on television, sponsored by law firms, warning of problems caused by pelvic mesh. Some pelvic mesh products were, indeed, withdrawn from the market. The products I use, when necessary, are all approved and still available.

Hysterectomy—Yes or No?

When the uterus hangs out of the vagina, a hysterectomy (removal of the uterus) may be an option. However, the vaginal tissue at the top of the vagina (where the uterus used to be) is then at risk of prolapsing.

During graduate medical training, I was taught to routinely do a hysterectomy with pelvic prolapse surgery. The thought process was that a falling uterus would continue to pull on any repair done to the bladder and rectum and compromise the repair in the long run. Now, more times than not, I return a normal uterus to its proper position and use the tough connective tissue of the cervix as one of my anchor points to place my stitches.

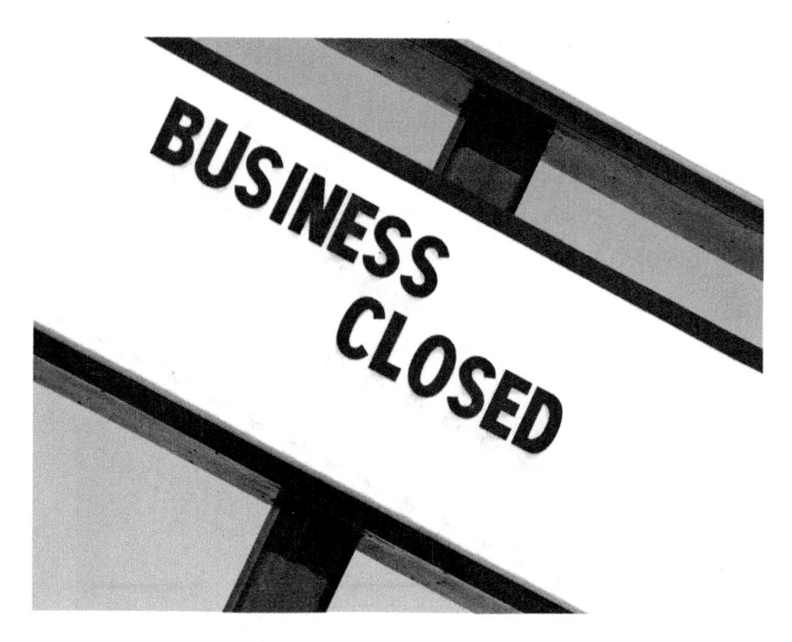

Colpocleisis—Shut It Down for Business

Finally, let me tell you about colpocleisis, a surgical procedure that is reserved for those women who never intend to have sex again. Simply stated, the surgeon permanently closes the inside walls of the vagina. From the outside everything looks like normal anatomy, but the length of the remaining vagina will only be about one inch. Anything that is inserted will run into a new wall.

> **Coming to Terms**
>
> ***Colpocleisis*** is a surgical procedure that permanently closes the inside walls of the vagina.

I know, I know—after your last delivery, maybe you felt like asking the doctor to just go ahead and sew that thing shut so that you'd never have to go through childbirth again. But that's not what this procedure is for.

A Humane Option

Surgically closing the vagina sounds extreme, and it is. But there are times when a colpocleisis is the most appropriate surgical management. For women with severe medical problems that make them unsuitable candidates for a restorative surgery, this procedure may be just what the doctor ordered.

Remember this picture?

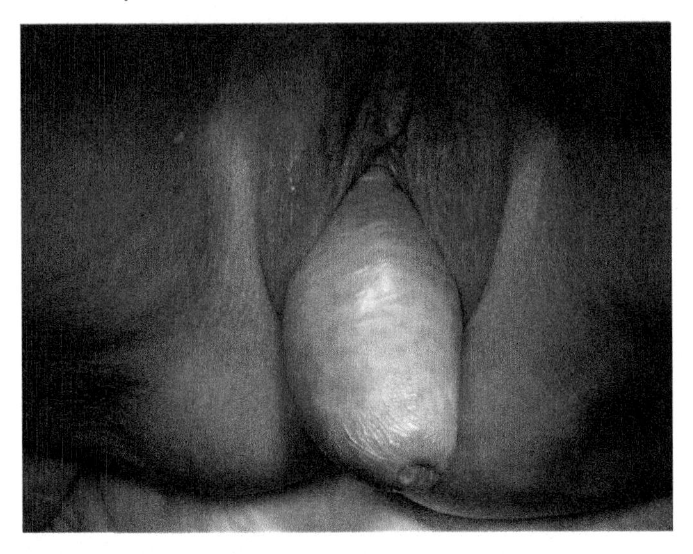

Now let's imagine this lady is eighty years old and in a nursing home. Every time she moves, her uterus slides on out of her vagina for a breath of air. A pessary causes ulcerations, or it won't stay in. She actually can't pee because the urethra bends 180 degrees in the wrong direction. Doomed to diapers again. With local anesthesia and light sedation, we can push her pelvic organs back into their proper place, and then sew her vagina shut to keep them there. For this lady, a colpocleisis would be a blessing.

Enough Description; It's Time to Wake Up

Whether your surgery was nip and tuck or more difficult, when I'm finished, it will be time for you to be taken to the recovery room. You'll stay there until you are fully awake, and if you're staying, you'll be transferred to a room.

Hospital Stay

Pelvic repairs often require an overnight stay in the hospital. The long-acting local anesthetic in the nerve block I gave you will keep you comfortable for the first eighteen to twenty-four hours after surgery.

Pelvic repairs often require an overnight hospital stay.

You'll have a ***catheter*** (a thin plastic tube) to drain urine from your bladder, and I may order a drip in your arm to replenish fluids.

You will notice a long piece of white gauze, which was placed in your vagina to help prevent bleeding. It will be removed the morning following surgery. Your stitches will usually dissolve on their own after a few weeks.

Prevent Constipation

This topic might seem trivial, but it's not. It is important for you to prevent constipation during your post-operative recovery period. You don't want to endure excessive pain with defecation or risk ripping out your stitches down there, compromising your repair.

You do not need to have a bowel movement before leaving the hospital. However, I would like for you to have one at home by the end of the next day. The pain medications that you will be taking can slow your gut down. To prevent constipation, you may begin taking a stool softener ahead of your surgery and do what you would normally do to keep regular. I will give you an instruction sheet with steps that help prevent adverse outcomes resulting from constipation. In the instructions, I outline steps to take if you have not had a bowel movement after breakfast on your second day home from the hospital.

Post Surgery

Although the recovery process is different for everyone, as a general rule you can expect to be up and walking around within a day after your surgery. You may shower on the day following surgery, but no tub baths for at least four weeks.

Be sure to take your pain medication as directed. You should anticipate some bruising and swelling, which might linger for as long as two to four weeks. Some patients experience vaginal bleeding similar to a light menstrual period or some vaginal discharge for a few weeks. During this time, do not insert tampons. Instead, use sanitary napkins or panty liners.

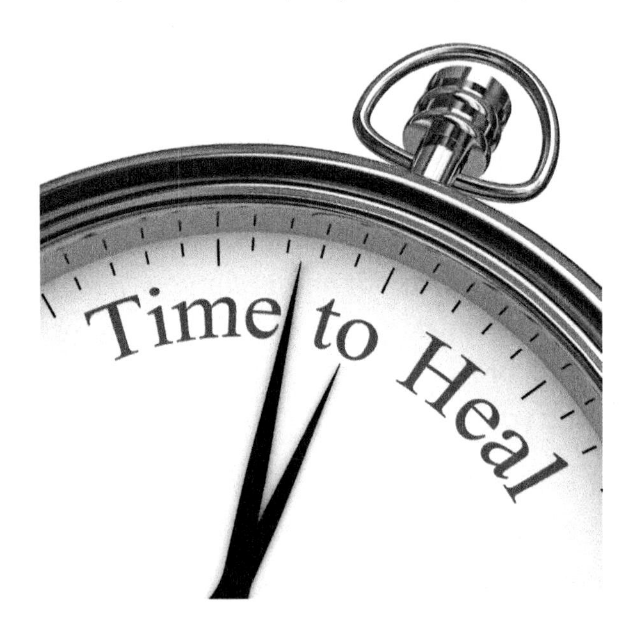

Heal and Recover

Now is the time for you to heal and recover. Take it easy; avoid stress to your treated area. Start slowly and increase your activity level gradually. For about a month, you'll want to avoid vigorous physical activities. No jogging or bouncing for up to six weeks.

Increase your activity level gradually.

Returning to work will depend on how strenuous that would be for you. Allow yourself enough time to rest, so that when you do return to work, you won't jeopardize your healing process.

And What about Sex?

Wait six weeks before you resume sex. When you begin having sex again, you will have to go gently with those inner tissues because you will be tight and tender inside. You will find more advice on this topic in chapter nine, "Toying with Sex."

Looking Ahead to a Bright Future

Won't it be wonderful to face the future without the discomfort and worrisome symptoms you used to experience before having your pelvic problem fixed?

Now you face a wonderful future.

Now is the time to give some thought to controlling any activities that might have contributed to your prolapse. You should avoid heavy lifting, long periods of standing, or other activities that put strain on your lower pelvic muscles.

Pay attention to your health. Stay at a weight that is healthy for you; avoid constipation; and of course, for your best health, no smoking.

You Are a Sexy New Woman

Well, we've come to the end of "Part Two: Now What Happens?" Leaving behind all those Granny Vagina Dilemmas we've talked about thus far, you should be ready and eager to start enjoying an active, satisfying sex life again.

You are a sexy new woman, but in my practice I've discovered there are some pressing sexual issues that even sexy new women are reluctant to talk about. So next, I'm including four chapters of personal topics I've titled "Part Three: The HUSH-HUSH Section."

Part

Three

The Hush-Hush Section

Chapter Six

Yo Thang be Raggedy

Warning

The following four chapters contain material that may not be suitable for male readers. Caution is advised. If a man should approach while you have this section open and ask, "What are you reading?" just flip to another section and say, "Oh, just woman stuff, nothing you'd be interested in."

Granny Vagina Dilemma: "We don't talk about that."

There are some things women are reluctant to talk about, even with each other. But what if life resembled that popular movie where everyone had to be honest, and once a group of women let their guard down, they all had to tell the truth about their vaginas. Wouldn't that situation be interesting?

So, let's make up a story—one that never happened, probably never will—but a fun story, nonetheless.

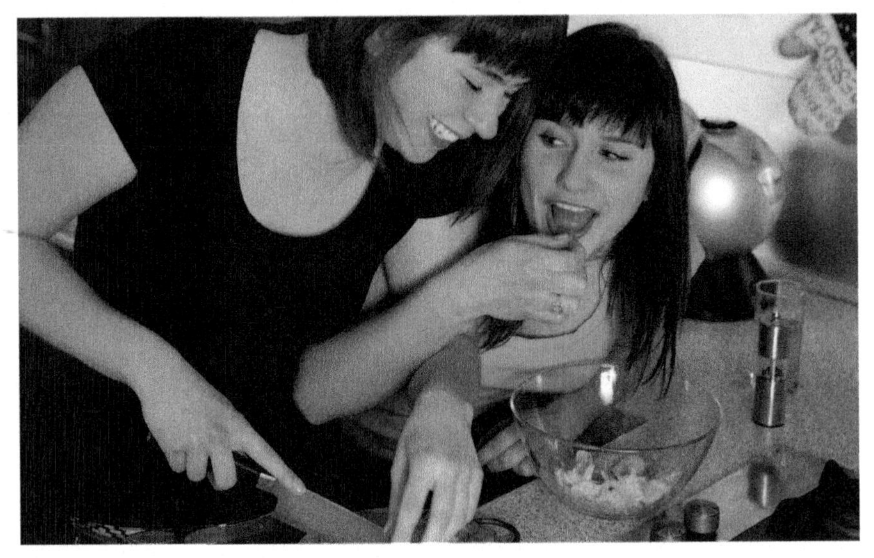

Here's our make-believe scene: a group of women were preparing food and chatting together while their husbands and significant others were watching a football game on television in another room. Suddenly, the women's conversation took an unexpected turn:

Vagina Doctor

"We understand you're the vagina doctor."

Preparations for the post-game cookout were underway. I was bustling around my friend's kitchen, juggling a glass of wine and unwrapping relish trays, trying to keep the olives from rolling onto the floor.

Two women had wandered into the kitchen in search of me. At the sound of the "v" word, the rest of the kitchen crew looked up, gave the newcomers the once-over-lightly, then looked away with only a barely discernible pause—the universal woman-signal that, although they might appear uninterested in what's about to come, they're curious, definitely curious and listening with both ears.

The newcomers glanced at each other nervously. In spite of their embarrassment, it was clear they thought I was going to be able to solve a problem for them.

"Can you make someone tighter?" the bolder one asked, her voice hushed almost to a whisper.

I wasn't exactly sure what she was referring to. "Well, sure," I ventured. "Vagina tightening is one of my favorite surgeries."

Silence descended over the countertops. As if on cue, food preparation was abandoned. Serious talk was best conducted with drinks in hand.

"So," I went on, "does this person have a problem?"

The questioner glanced at the other women in the room, determined not to retreat now that she had come this far. Again, the hushed voice. "She thinks she does."

I was just about to give my standard caveat—I don't discuss patients' problems in public—but I didn't have a chance to get another word in edgewise.

Before I could open my mouth, the second newcomer, who had been letting her friend speak for her, faced her audience and blurted, "Your husbands are about the same age as mine. Do they fall out when you try to make love? My husband calls me his cave woman. He says I'm like a cavern in there."

This confession struck a sympathetic chord with the salad lady. "Yeah, it's no fun when your man always flips out." The speaker paused, then blushed, realizing she had just revealed a secret about her own sex life. She looked around defensively. "I suppose none of you are as big as a bucket?"

Someone shouted, "I'm so big that I can't keep tampons in."

Someone else did her one better. Waving around a tiny sausage, she squealed, "I'm so big that having sex is like sliding a hot dog down a hallway!"

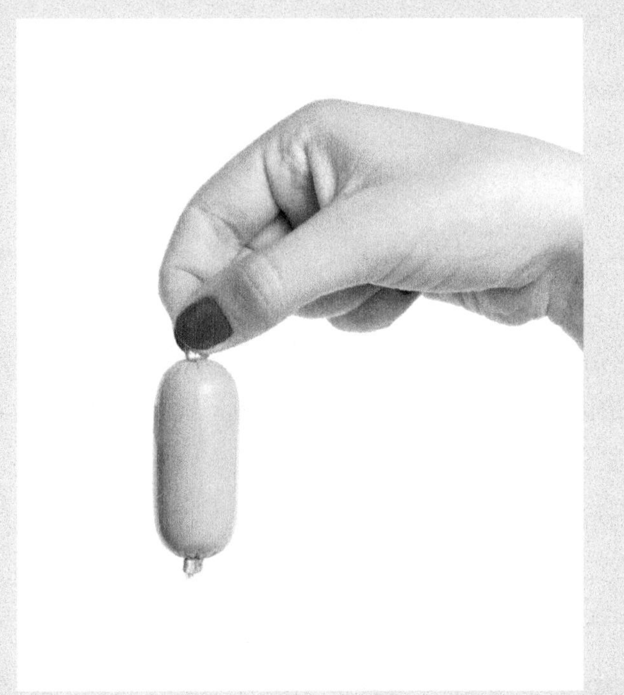

Whereupon her neighbor hissed in the hot dog lady's ear, "Well, when I get wet down there, my man has to tie a board to his butt to keep from falling in."

It seems we had hit upon a topic of universal concern.

Out of the corner of my eye I noticed my friend's elderly aunt, who considered herself in command of the kitchen. She winced. Were things getting out of hand here?

"Oh dear," I murmured. "Now we've offended Aunt Emma."

Briskly, Aunt Emma refilled her wine glass, moved over to the sink and turned on the faucet. Wetting her palms, she pressed them together and began making loud smacking sounds. She continued until she had everyone's attention.

"Hear that? Twat farts," she said. "That's what we called them in my day, twat farts."

"Every time my Henry stuck his thing in me, he pushed air out my twat and it made a noise. Scared him at first, but he got used to it over the years. Let me tell you, when his engine got revved up, it sounded like a gun fight going on down there between my legs."

The room erupted, women all trying to talk at once. Pandemonium. Chaos. What's not to like?

A few men gingerly peeped around the kitchen door as if expecting to see a bear thrashing its way across the room. Of course, it took some fast talking to assure the menfolk they needn't call 9-1-1. "Just get back in front of the television, guys. Yes, yes, we'll have the food ready by the end of the game."

Granny Vagina Dilemma: "What if he thinks I'm raggedy?"

That last story may have come from our imagination, but in real life it's natural for women to worry about what their menfolk are going to say about their saggy, baggy vaginas. Here's a story of something that actually happened:

Real Men Don't Poke Fun

After a rap concert at a local Aspen venue, a group of us fans stood around the edge of the stage. We were in good spirits, enjoying the rollicking atmosphere, along with the band's bodyguard. Picture this scene: the bodyguard was at least 6'3", a 350-pound imposing man with gold chains down to his knees; but as it turned out, he was a gentle giant.

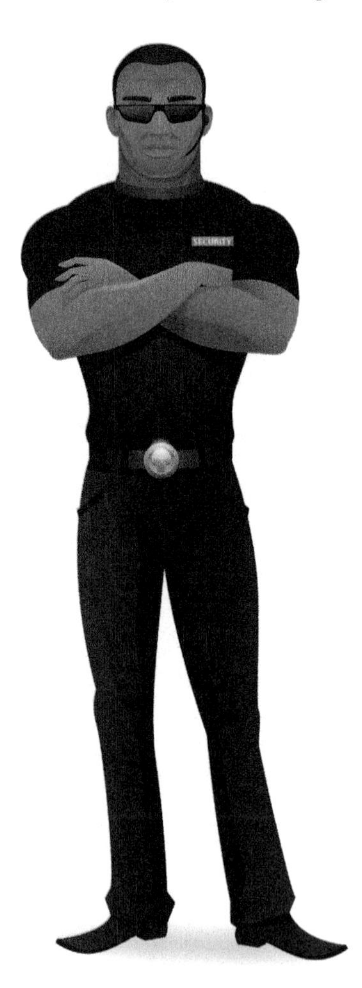

When our conversation turned to what I do for a living, vaginas came up, of course. I described how I help women with their saggy, baggy Granny Vaginas. The bodyguard laughed. Then I mentioned that their husbands often thanked me afterwards. This idea caught his attention.

He said he always thought it was the man's job to see to it his woman was satisfied in bed, and went on to say he would never hurt his woman's feelings. "I'm serious," he said. "What am I supposed to say to her? Hey, yo thang be raggedy! You need to get that thang fixed."

Even men from macho backgrounds are sensitive to their women's feelings. The bodyguard would never call his woman raggedy, and in a loving relationship, your man isn't going to call you raggedy, either.

Vagina and Vulva Are Not the Same

"What am I supposed to say to her? Hey, yo thang be raggedy! You need to get that thang fixed."

If we don't call it "Yo Thang," what shall we call it? Two terms—***vagina*** and ***vulva***—are often used interchangeably, but they're not the same.

Coming to Terms

Vagina—Your ***vagina*** is inside you. It is a hollow tube about three to seven inches long, extending from your uterus to its entrance down there between your legs. You may refer to your vagina as the "***birth canal***" because it is the passageway through which a baby travels as it is born.

The opening to your vagina is called, appropriately enough, your ***vaginal opening***, and the small chamber just inside your vaginal opening is your ***introitus.***

Vulva—Your ***vulva*** refers to the external female genitalia surrounding your vaginal opening. You can see all the parts of your vulva outside your body. We'll give your vulva center stage in the next chapter.

Your Questions

As I was saying before all hell broke loose in our kitchen story, there are some things women are reluctant to talk about—even with each other. Unless the setting is right. Let's go back and continue with our make-believe. By now the women in the kitchen have calmed down. My friends have returned to their food preparation tasks with wine glasses close at hand. The setting is right, and I'm being peppered with questions:

"So, Dr. King, just what is the right tight?"

I hold up two fingers, close together. Ideally, your vagina's interior diameter should be small enough to allow for comfortable penetration by two fingers (about the size of a man's penis when he's aroused). You want to be tight enough so that you get stimulated, too. Inside there, your tissue should be flexible but not floppy.

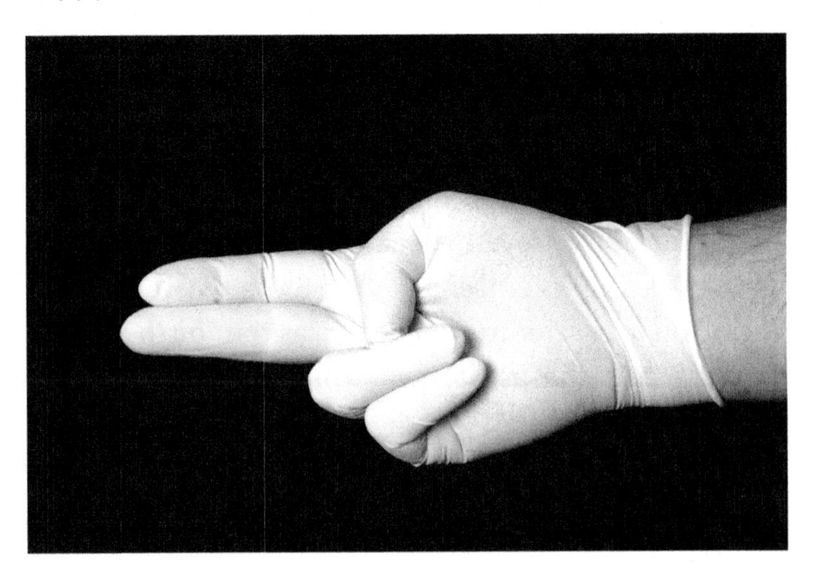

You want to be tight enough so that you get stimulated, too.

If you're not two-fingers tight ... well, as I said, vagina tightening is one of my favorite surgeries.

"And who gets themselves tightened? Just movie stars?"

Think about the progression of a relationship. When we're dating, we want to put our best foot forward: we fix our hair and makeup, we wear flattering and fashionable clothes, and we're polite and considerate of each other's feelings. After we make a commitment, we want to please our new partner.

Life goes on. We have children together, and those children anchor us as a family.

As the relationship matures, the children grow and demand less of our attention. It's time to renew and refresh the commitment you made with your mate. At this point, it isn't fair to simply let yourself go. Perhaps it's time to get your vagina tightened and add some "Boo-Yah to your Hoo-Hah."

Perhaps it's time to add some "Boo-Yah to your Hoo-Hah."

In this country today, tightening is not uncommon among women whose husbands are famous sports figures. These wives come to me to get their vaginas tightened after they have babies, because other "sports wives" are doing it.

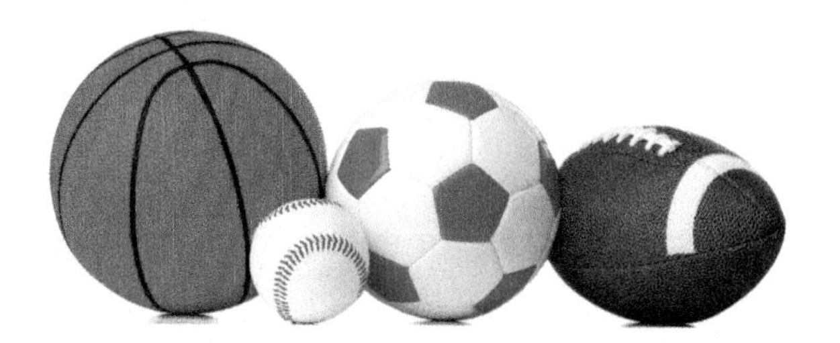

But they're not the only ones. Most women in my practice who are undergoing a pelvic repair also choose to include vaginal tightening at the same time. If you are going to get fixed, don't stop half way.

If you're going to get fixed, don't stop half way.

Now let's think about it from your own standpoint. If I should ask you, "Do you want to be loose or do you want to be tight?" I'll bet you would all prefer a nice pre-baby-tight vagina. Wouldn't it be great to go back to the way you were before you had kids? Do you even remember what that was like?

"Why didn't my vagina just snap back in shape after having kids?"

Some women do. But many women's vaginas don't return to their pre-pregnancy state. Your vagina has to stretch out extremely far to let that baby pass. Sometimes your vaginal canal gets torn, or the tissue breaks down, so that your vagina can end up saggy and baggy. Vaginal birth can cause nerve and muscle damage, which over time just gets worse.

Other things can happen, too. The ***perineal body*** (the muscular area right outside the bottom of your vaginal opening) can shorten and become thinner, even separate in the midline. Or maybe you had an ***episiotomy*** (a fancy word for when the doctor makes an incision to enlarge the opening to your vagina so that it won't tear when the baby passes through).

Coming to Terms

Your ***perineal body*** is the muscular area right outside the bottom of your vaginal opening.

An ***episiotomy*** is an incision to enlarge the opening to the vagina.

Then you have more pregnancies, more deliveries. Soon, as the lady in our story said, you end up being his cave woman.

Think about what happens when a man stretches a condom over his erect penis. Five minutes later (okay, let's be generous and say thirty minutes later) does that condom return to its original shape? No. It stays stretched out. The same thing happens each time your vaginal canal gets stretched; it loses some of its elasticity.

"I haven't had any children, but I think I'm really big inside."

Nature didn't give all of us the same size vaginas. Some women are just naturally big and baggy in there. Or something else can affect it, like smoking or gaining and losing weight.

When you go home tonight, do the two-finger test. If you're way too loose in there, you may be missing out on pleasure.

"I thought Kegels were supposed to tighten you up."

You know what? Doing exercises to tighten an unhealthy, stretched out vagina is an urban myth. Way back in the 1940s, a doctor named Kegel developed some squeezing exercises (which we now refer to as ***Kegels***) to help women who had problems with loss of urine. Some of those patients reported their sex life improved, and ever since then women are being told they can Kegel their way to tighter sex.

Unfortunately, Kegel exercises can't repair significant injuries to your vaginal muscles and tissue. If your vagina is otherwise healthy, I recommend you try them, as exercises can improve vaginal muscle tone. But you'll probably find that doing Kegels is more frustrating than effective for tightening an over-stretched, damaged vagina.

"Do you have something better to offer than Kegels?"

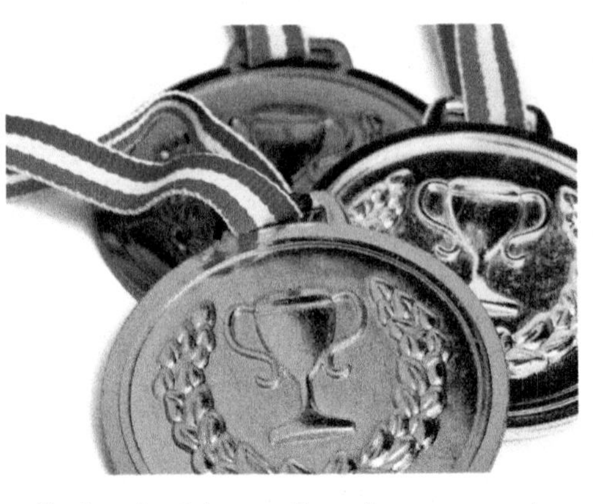

I sure do. I've completed training in a new method of using laser surgery to tighten and support the vagina. As I do vaginal surgery, I use sutures to pull the inside walls of your vagina together to make it as tight as you wish. Then I add a final step, injecting platelet-rich-plasma along the suture lines to promote rapid healing.

Kegeling is not an Olympic sport!

"But will my tight va jay jay last?"

My goal is for your repair to be a lasting one; I do not mean for this surgery to be just a temporary solution. Your vagina and its supporting structures will be restored to a more youthful, pre-pregnancy state.

My goal is for your repair to be a lasting one.

Keep in mind, however, that there are many factors outside my control that might affect an individual's long-term results: age, health of tissue being treated, future childbearing, chronic coughing, or pelvic injuries, for example.

And So, Ladies, Aren't You Glad We Had This Little Talk?

- If you thought there was no solution for your "big as a bucket" vagina,
- If you thought your cavernous crotch was just a part of aging, and
- If you didn't know where to go for help ...

Now you know, a solution is possible.

Coming Up Next

Next, in the second of our four HUSH-HUSH chapters, we'll discuss a problem that women find even more embarrassing than a gaping vagina—so embarrassing that they're often afraid to admit it to their gynecologist!

Chapter Seven

The Aesthetically Challenged Vulva

Your Vulva

Although your external genitals (visible outer parts of your sex organs) are commonly referred to as vagina, your vagina is the "birth canal," and it is up inside you where you can't see it. The correct term for the part that covers and protects the vaginal opening, visible from the outside, is your vulva.

What You See Is What You've Got—But We Can Change All That

"I'm embarrassed to say this but ..."

Let me begin this chapter with the true-to-life story of a patient who came to me with a problem—a very personal problem she had suffered with from her teen years through adulthood; but she had never, ever, had the nerve to breathe a word about it to anyone.

As is typical for many women with her Dilemma, she made an appointment for an annual exam—a way to approach me without getting right down to the most pressing issue that she had always been afraid to bring up with any other doctor.

When I finished her exam, I asked my standard questions: "Is there anything else? Is sex tight enough?"

My patient hesitated; nervously, she said sex was all right, although she had to squeeze during sex to make it tight enough. Then, taking a deep breath, she confided:

"I'm embarrassed to say this, but I don't like the way I look down there."

"I don't like the way I look down there."

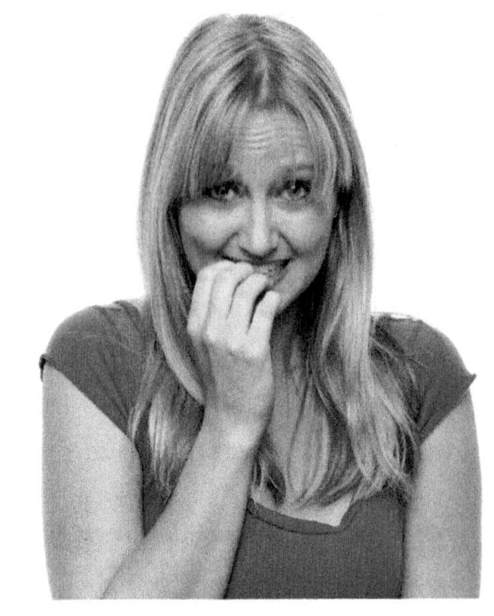

I always admire women who can overcome what, for them, is terrible embarrassment when talking about their genital area.

My goal is to create a safe, non-threatening atmosphere in the privacy of my office. Seriously and gently I asked, "When did it start?"

She said that, when she was a teenager and first started her menstrual periods, her outer folds of skin "down there" began to grow bigger—and then they just grew and grew.

Although her tissue was healthy and not diseased, the outer part of her genital area (labia) had, indeed, grown into large, unsightly flaps.

Coming to Terms

The folds of the vulva that surround a woman's or girl's genital organs are called ***labia***. The medical term for overgrowth of labia is ***labial hypertrophy***.

I handed her a mirror. "Let me show you what I'm seeing and you can tell me what you don't like," I said. She indicated how self-conscious she felt about her overgrown labia. Then, while she looked in the mirror, I took a Q-Tip and pushed the skin of her vulva smooth and taunt, showing what most women like to have done when I surgically correct this condition.

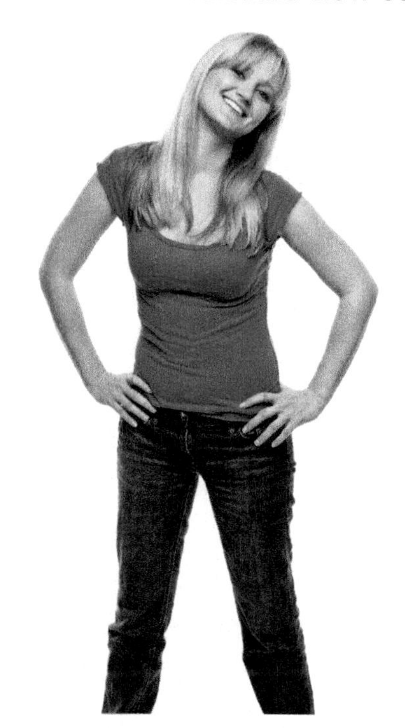

By the time my patient left, she was relaxed and smiling. Happy she had come in, happy someone was listening. Relieved that she did not feel she was being judged or trivialized.

When I told her I was writing a book for women that would explain labial surgery, she urged, "You do need to write a book so that women can find out about it. Please write that book. Women need to be educated."

And so, Gentle Readers, here's everything you ever wanted to know about labial surgery but were afraid to ask.

Coming to Terms

Labioplasty (also known as ***labiaplasty*** and ***labial reduction***) is a cosmetic surgery procedure for altering the inner and outer lips (folds of skin) surrounding a woman's vulva.

What it is not: Surgery to re-sculpt and beautify your vulva is ***NOT female circumcision***, which would be to remove the hood of the ***clitoris***, the small sexual organ at the top of the vaginal opening.

Your Vulva Has Labia ("Lips")

Your labia's two rounded folds of fatty tissue are the ***labia majora***. They are the hair-bearing, slightly darker-colored skin along the outer surfaces of your labia. Between them are two flat reddish folds of inner tissue called ***labia minora***. Most people refer to the labia minora as the "lips."

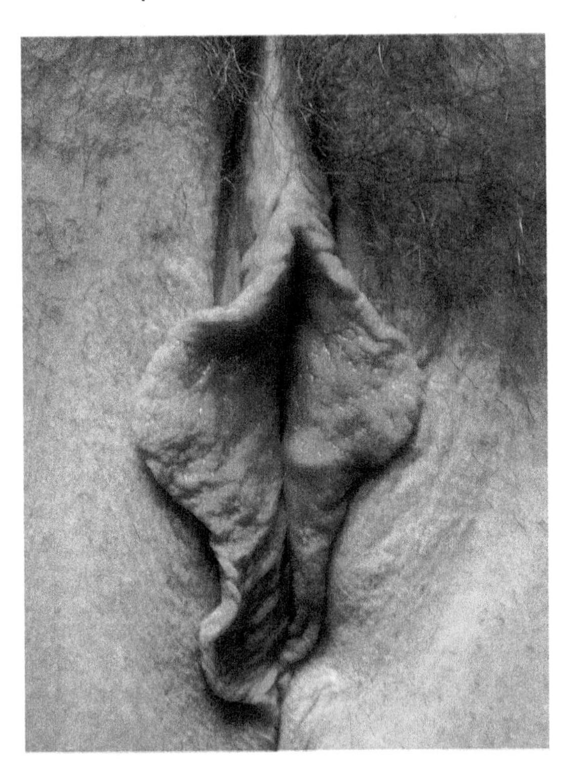

As we shall see, these lips can vary greatly in size from woman to woman. You could be blessed with labia that are smooth and perky the way they are portrayed in girlie magazine pictures. Or you could suffer terrible embarrassment because

- they are overly long or thick;
- they are uneven or lopsided;
- they are discolored; or
- you think they are downright ugly.

How Did Your Labia Get to Be the Way They Are?

They Just Grew That Way

Maybe your outsized labia grew large of their own accord.

You might have been born with a tendency toward fast-growing, larger-than-normal inner lips. But for most women, labial growth takes place gradually. From their early-childhood size, labia begin growing longer in puberty as your body readies itself for reproduction. During pregnancy or immediately afterwards, labia tend to grow even more. Your inner and outer labia may not grow evenly on each side of your vulva, and they may not stop growing until they are so large that they cause problems.

During pregnancy, labia tend to grow.

Outside Influences

Other things can affect the shape and condition of your labia, as well. They may become saggy around menopause, or they may grow larger or smaller as you gain and lose weight. And of course, they're often subjected to stretching and trauma.

Childbirth

Childbirth (need I tell you?) takes its toll on your vulva. Those tissues have to stretch way out to allow the baby to pass. Sometimes they can't stretch far enough, allowing a cut or tear that does not heal properly. I've seen big notches and actual holes in women's labia due to childbirth trauma.

Childbirth takes its toll on your vulva.

Five Areas of Concern

There are lots and lots of problems associated with your outer lady-parts. Some you've only heard about. Some you're intimately familiar with. And some you only talk about in HUSH-HUSH tones. Basically, there are five areas of concern: (1) sex, (2) other women's opinions, (3) hygiene and comfort, (4) wardrobe malfunction, and (5)—underlying it all—your feelings of self-esteem.

In this chapter, we'll cover the whole wide range, but I know what's right up there at the top of your list: SEX. Good place to start. When an aesthetically challenged vulva keeps you from enjoying your sex life to its fullest, that is, indeed, a Dilemma.

> **Your Sex Partner**
>
> *In the context of our discussion, your "sex partner" is the person with whom you engage in sex. Gender of your sex partner is not the issue, nor is the type of relationship. Just for convenience, I'll refer to your sex partner as male.*

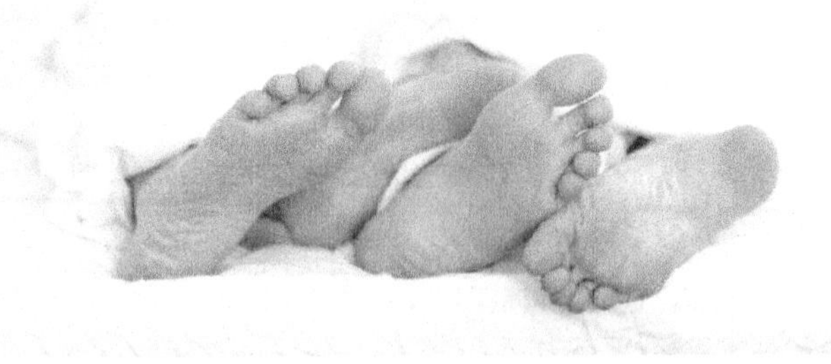

1. Sexual Issues

Ugly Vulva Dilemma: "Ouch! That hurts!"

Your sex partner might not even be aware of what's happening: his penis grabs your long labial flap, dragging it into your vagina.

One or both sides of your labia curl inward and move in and out, pinching with each thrust. Yes, that's painful!

Ugly Vulva Dilemma: "Oral sex? Oh, no!"

Maybe you can convince him oral sex is against your religion.

Ugly Vulva Dilemma: "Let's just turn out the lights."

What's a woman to do when she is ashamed to let her sex partner see what she looks like "down there" between her legs? Well, she could try to keep herself covered until she can turn out the lights. Several women have told me that their husbands have never seen them naked with the lights on.

Men don't understand why women are so bothered.

Although you may find your labia mortifying to the point of affecting your life, that might not be the way it is for your man. He probably still finds you very attractive. Generally, men don't get it; they don't understand why women are so bothered by the looks of their labia.

The point, however, is not what someone else thinks. The point is, if you're ashamed or embarrassed, then for you it is a massive problem.

Ugly Vulva Dilemma: "Good grief, he's seen me!"

How do men react when they see bat wings from hell down there? In my practice, I find that men who are in a loving relationship are eager to help their women feel confident and would never say anything cruel.

On the other hand, young men in casual relationships can be very insensitive. For instance, here is what one patient told me:

When she was in her early twenties, her boyfriend looked at her distended labia and said, "Oh my God, you must have had a lot of sex, look how long they are!" He was insinuating that she was promiscuous. This comment scarred her for decades. Even though she eventually entered into a loving marriage with a kind and caring spouse, she retained the negative image of herself brought on by that crass comment. It impacted her self-image during sex and made her self-conscious in not wanting her husband to see her naked. Happily, this lovely lady sought surgical correction and her self-esteem was restored.

There's an App for That

You don't need to give up, or miss out on the best possible sex because of the size and shape of your genitalia. As they say in the tech world "there's an app for that." With labial surgery—an elective, cosmetic procedure—we can design the vulva of your dreams. Then you'll be ready for your lover to take a good look and you will feel comfortable and not embarrassed.

Labial surgery can design the vulva of your dreams.

2. Other Women Don't Look This Way

We've talked about how embarrassing it is to be seen by men when your lady-parts are downright ugly, but the same embarrassment extends to being seen by other women.

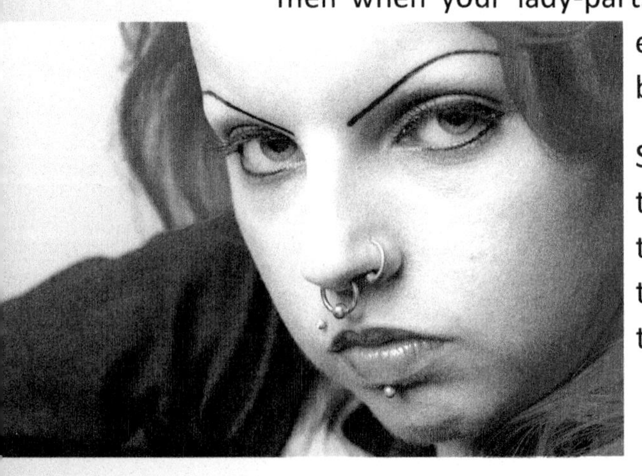

Some women go out of their way to be different from other women: they dye their hair, get piercings and tattoos, or wear clothing that makes them distinctive.

All these options are yours to make by choice. But you had no choice in the matter of the vulva that Mother Nature handed to you, and what if you don't like it?

Ugly Vulva Dilemma: "My sister teases me."

This Dilemma begins in your teenage years, when girls are apt to say cruel things to each other. Girls see each other naked from time to time (especially sisters or best friends). If your labia hang off you like a duck's bill, you can expect any girl who sees them to wince and say something wicked, even though you already know it looks weird, and you don't need someone to remind you.

Your labia may hang off you like a duck's bill.

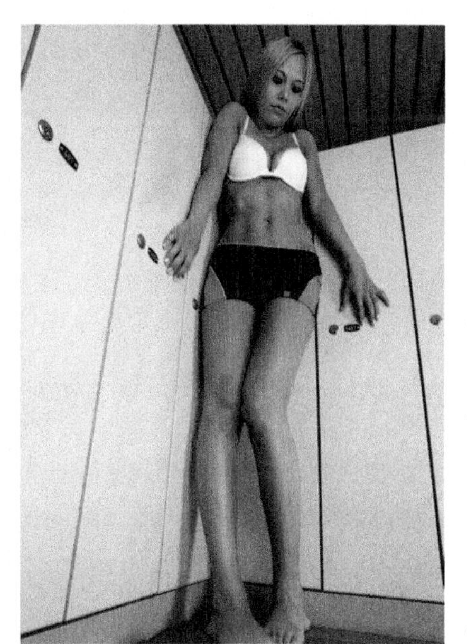

Ugly Vulva Dilemma: "I won't undress in the locker room."

Your swim class just finished, and all the women are heading for the locker room to peel off their wet suits. How many corners are there for you to hide in?

3. There Are Hygiene and Comfort Issues

To put it bluntly, you're risking your health with overly long, distorted labia. Extra folds of tissue become chafed, pinched, and painful. And if the condition is left uncorrected, you've created a haven for germs and bacteria to hide and multiply. One woman reported that the outer edges of her lips were dark and dirty looking, so that a man was afraid to have sex with her because he thought she had a disease.

Overly-long, distorted labia are a health risk.

Ugly Vulva Dilemma: "I have computer crotch."

Here's a new Dilemma brought on by today's phenomenon of sitting for long periods of time in front of a computer screen.

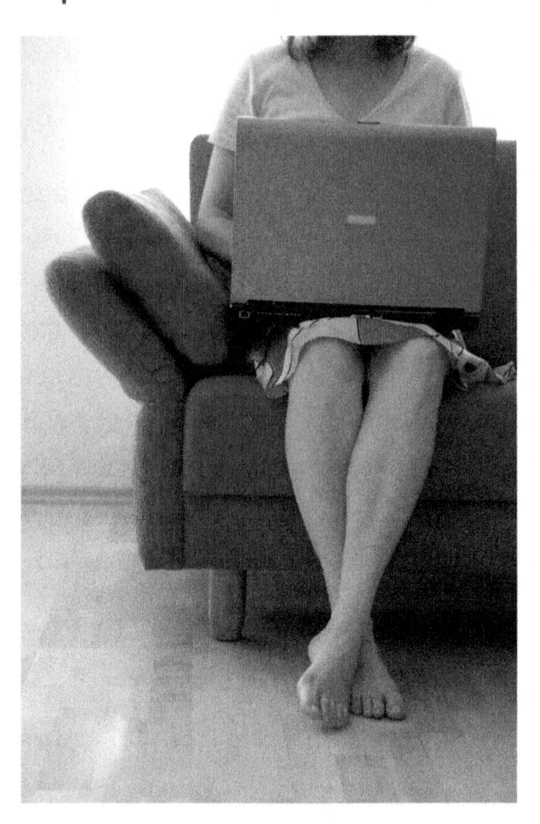

When your inner or outer lips (labia minora or labia majora) are so elongated that they extend well beyond the vaginal opening, they become compacted when you sit. The result: pain and irritation.

Ugly Vulva Dilemma: "I pee every which way."

Do you have a multi-directional urine stream? You know, like a lawn sprinkler. When all your lady-parts fit together as nature intended, your labia should help direct a steady stream, not deflect urine all over you and the toilet seat.

Ugly Vulva Dilemma: "What's that odor? Good grief, it's me!"

Women whose labia are distended worry that they can't keep themselves as clean as they would like. When this Dilemma happens, odor develops. Smelly yeast infections and even bacterial infections can occur within the folds to cause itching and burning.

4. Wardrobe Malfunction

This problem's not limited to famous singers and movie stars. When any woman's vulva is flabby, saggy, baggy, or lumpy, she is limited to a wardrobe that doesn't broadcast her generous genital condition to the world.

Not limited to famous singers and movie stars.

Ugly Vulva Dilemma: "Thong? Wrong!"

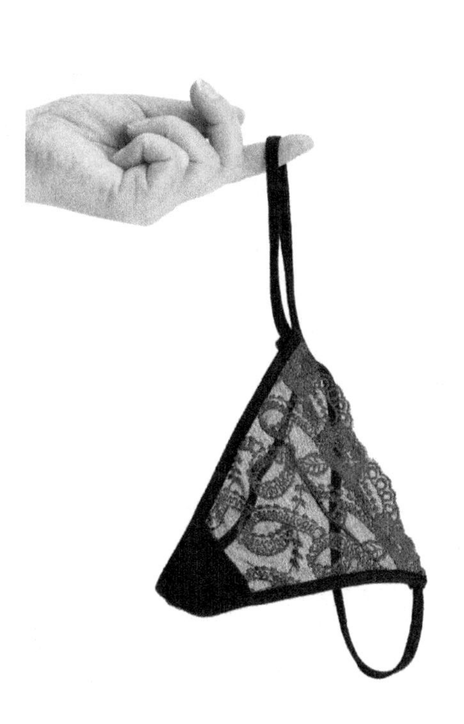

They may be all the rage for other women, but underwear thongs are totally off limits for you if your labia would come hanging out the edges. Just hike on over to the lingerie department and buy yourself some granny bloomers.

Ugly Vulva Dilemma: "No, that's not a scrotum in my swimsuit."

Oh sure, we would all like to look smooth and tight like ballerinas down there. But if your labial lips are too fat and bulging, they're going to create a big bulge between your legs—a bulge that will look as if you're carrying around a man's scrotum.

Pass on that cute teeny-weeny-bikini.

So, you will have to pass on that cute teeny-weeny-bikini and go for the swimsuit with the ample panty bottom, hoping and praying you'll be able to keep everything tucked in.

Ugly Vulva Dilemma: "I got a bikini wax and now everything shows."

You used to count on your genital hair to provide sort of a camouflage for your ugly labia. A bikini wax bares all.

Ugly Vulva Dilemma: "My crack looks like a camel toe."

I remember the day another surgeon called me and said, "Someone's asked if I can take care of camel toe. Do you know what that is?"

"Camel toe" is a popular term for what happens when the pants (or swimsuit or shorts) you're wearing ride up so tight between your legs that they create a cavernous crack up the middle of your genitals. (Check out camel toe on the Internet to see lots of pictures illustrating what it looks like.)

Coming to Terms

"***Camel toe***" happens when the pants (or swimsuit or shorts) you're wearing ride up so tight between your legs that they create a cavernous crack up the middle of your genitals.

Why's It Called Camel Toe?

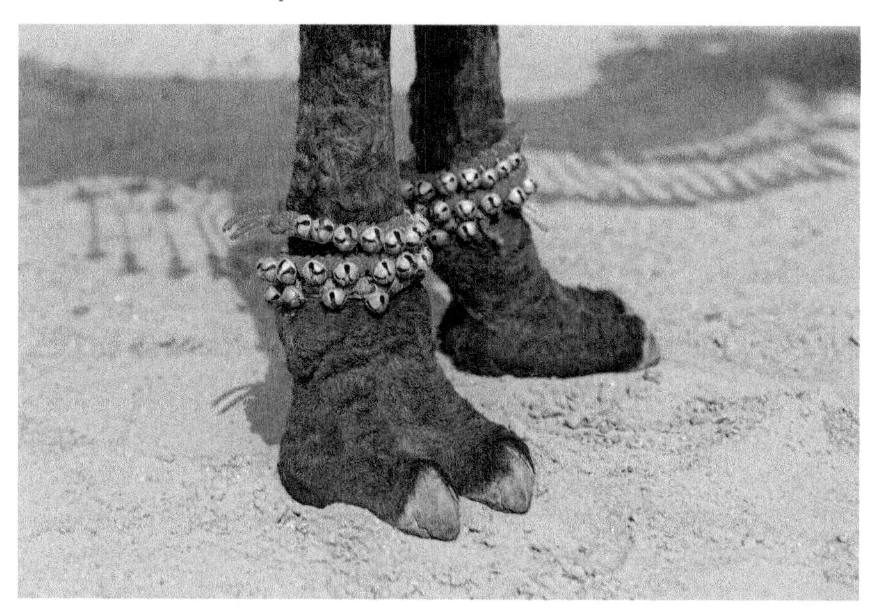

Camels have toes that are split in the middle. It helps them walk in the sand. Nice for camels, but not much fun for you when people make fun of your split. Of course, some girls want to look that way. They wear their pants too tight and think it's sexy.

But if you are wearing normal clothes and you have too much fat or too much saggy skin in your labia majora (outer lips), so that they bulge out (and you don't want to look like a camel toe), then cosmetic surgery can reduce your labia back to normal size.

5. Self-Esteem: "I don't like the way I look down there."

Self-esteem underlies all these problems.

Now that we've discussed sex, other women's opinions, hygiene, and wardrobe concerns, let's turn to the universal issue underlying all these problems: your self-esteem.

Remember my patient who nervously confided, ***"I'm embarrassed to say this, but I don't like the way I look down there."***

Embarrassed

Why are so many women embarrassed to admit that they're displeased with the way their genitalia look?

Are Women Afraid to Talk about Sex?

Admittedly, sex was once a taboo subject, but these days most of us are relatively comfortable talking about sex. There's something more going on here.

The Clue

We'll find the clue in my patient's response after she and I had openly discussed her feelings about her overgrown labia. She was relieved because her fear of being humiliated had not materialized; she was not being judged or trivialized for wanting to do something about her appearance down there.

Judge Not—Trivialize Not

In our society, there are nay-sayers who are quick to pass negative judgment before they know all the facts (condemnation before investigation).

Furthermore, we still find nay-sayers clinging to the old-fashioned notion that doing something for the purpose of boosting your own self-esteem is foolish, not to mention futile, and certainly to be frowned upon.

Attitudes Have Come a Long Way, Baby

Some of you may be old enough to remember this situation: about thirty years ago, when facial cosmetic surgery was starting to catch on in a big way, a woman had to present a valid (non-vanity) reason to justify her request for a face lift.

First, she had to pass a quiz: "Why do you want this procedure done?" A woman who replied "I want to look prettier," or—heaven forbid—"I want to feel better about myself," would be shown the door. Doctors felt ethically bound not to perform cosmetic surgery for those reasons. There was an attitude that, if a woman was suffering from a poor self-image, then cosmetic intervention would not do anything to alleviate the issue, and she would end up still suffering from a poor self-image. She should just go see a psychiatrist.

And There's Still a Way to Go

A negative attitude still persists in regard to labial surgery. When I first introduced the procedure, a nurse was heard scoffing at the idea: "I don't understand why anyone would have this done." Unfortunately, my patient, being prepped for the surgery, overheard that unprofessional remark. Nevertheless, she wanted her labia fixed, and after the surgery she was incredibly thrilled.

When I learned about the nurse's rude remark, I asked her whether she would have said that about a patient who was having a rhinoplasty (nose job) or a breast reduction. Fortunately, by now this nurse and most other nurses have been won over to the idea that surgery to correct unsightly or problematic labia is a positive experience. With new nurses I still have to start from scratch, taking care to explain the patient's decision to alter her appearance to something that makes her feel better about herself.

On My Soapbox Here

As a concerned physician, here is my opinion: when a woman believes she has a problem, we, as a society, should not trivialize, invalidate, or devalue her opinion by saying it's not a problem. It's not our place to tell her how she should or shouldn't feel because, bottom line, she actually does feel that way.

And she should be able to do something about her problem if she wishes. It's not up to you or me to make that value judgment.

My patients have valid concerns about their own bodies, and if they want something fixed, then it is strictly their decision to make. They deserve a well-thought-out, well-executed response, and a skilled surgeon with an aesthetic eye. I take pride in helping each of my patients attain a better, healthier "self."

Think about Breast Size

Labia come in many shapes and sizes; as with breasts, Mother Nature did not design them all the same. Picture yourself walking into the lingerie section of a department store to check out the bras. There are racks and racks of different sizes. Regular size bras for regular size breasts. Minimizer bras for women who think their breasts are too large. Padded bras for women who think their breasts are too small. (A well-known advice columnist used to say, "Fill in with cotton what nature's forgotten.")

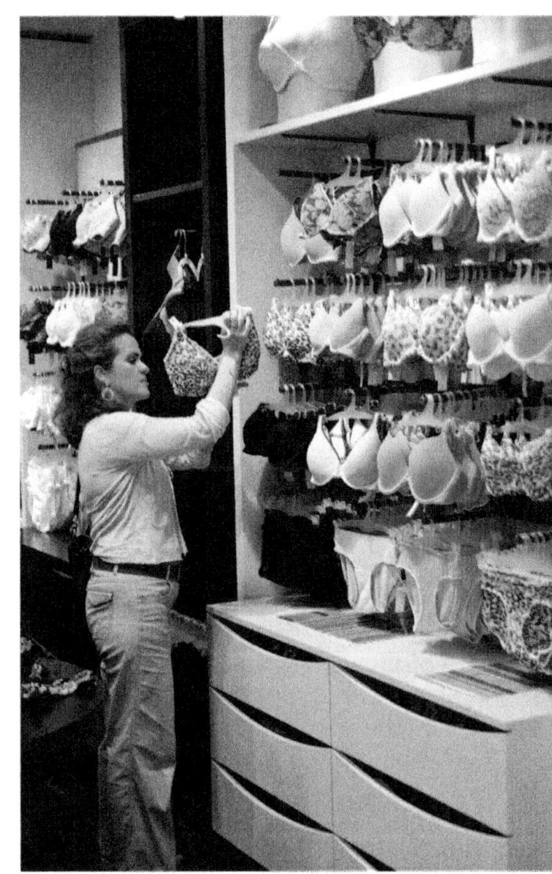

There are surgical procedures to reduce large

breasts, surgical procedures to augment small breasts, and surgical procedures to lift saggy, droopy breasts. Often these alterations are not medically necessary, but they serve a personal preference. Women seem to want to feel their best in their own skin.

Women want to feel their best in their own skin.

Interestingly, studies reveal how women react after breast augmentation. When they had flat chests, these women chose clothes to cover and hide themselves. After corrective surgery, they had an uplift in personality and became more self-confident. They were not embarrassed to wear tight clothing. Self-esteem was boosted immensely.

That's exactly the positive change in attitude experienced by women who undergo corrective labial surgery.

Labial Surgery Patients Are Thrilled with the Results

Overall, labioplasty can create youthful and aesthetically appealing vulvas. Women who have had labial surgery procedures are thrilled with the results. The source of their terrible embarrassment is gone. Here's the proof of success: many of them are telling their friends. What was once a taboo subject for them is now something they can't wait to tell other women.

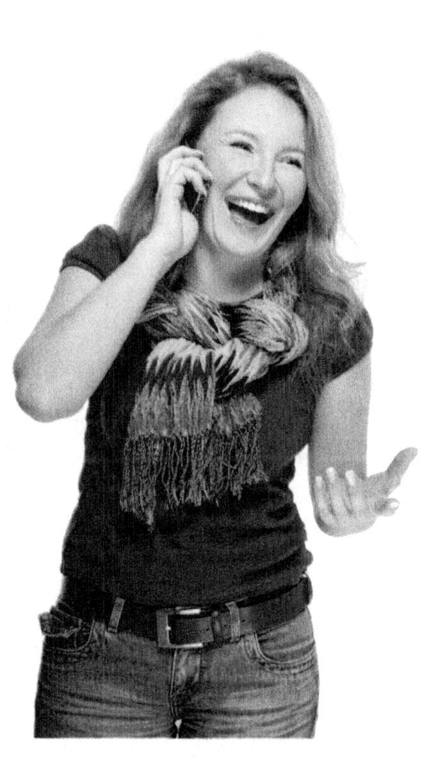

Now they can't wait to tell other women.

The Choice Is Yours, and Yours Alone, to Make

Maybe It's Not a Problem for You

Not everyone sees an ugly vulva as a Dilemma. If you're not bothered by the looks of your genital area, then it's not a problem. In fact, one of my patients has the ugliest vulva I have ever seen. Even I shudder to look at it. But, you know what? It doesn't bother her. To her it's not a problem. So, for me it's not a problem either. I am never, ever, the one to introduce the topic of changing the way your lady-parts look. We only talk about it if you bring up the subject.

But When You Say, "I don't like it ... "

On the other hand, there are women who come to my office having already decided they want surgery to correct the appearance of their labia. They begin the conversation by saying, "I don't like it. I want it changed." They are clear; they have an issue and they want it changed!

About the Procedure

Cutting and sculpting in the labial area is a delicate process. It is important to choose an experienced labioplasty surgeon who specializes in this procedure.

When I perform labioplasty, I use a laser surgery technique that is extremely gentle on labial tissue. After surgical enhancement of the vulva, I inject platelet-rich-plasma from each patient's own blood back along the suture lines to promote rapid healing.

A Sensible Solution

A problem with your labia is usually not life-threatening. Although cosmetic surgery in general, and labial surgery in particular, may not be necessary to sustain your physical existence, such procedures can certainly facilitate a higher quality of life. Having your ugly vulva made aesthetically pleasing is a safe, sensible solution that may be right for you.

Regarding Insurance

Labial restructuring, as well as vaginal tightening, are considered cosmetic procedures, and because they are not routine components of a pelvic repair, they are usually denied for insurance coverage.

Moving Right Along

Did you ever wish you could get your virginity back? Read on.

Chapter Eight

Hymen Hunting

In Aspen, Colorado, there is a special intersection between two streets: "Hyman" and "Hunter."

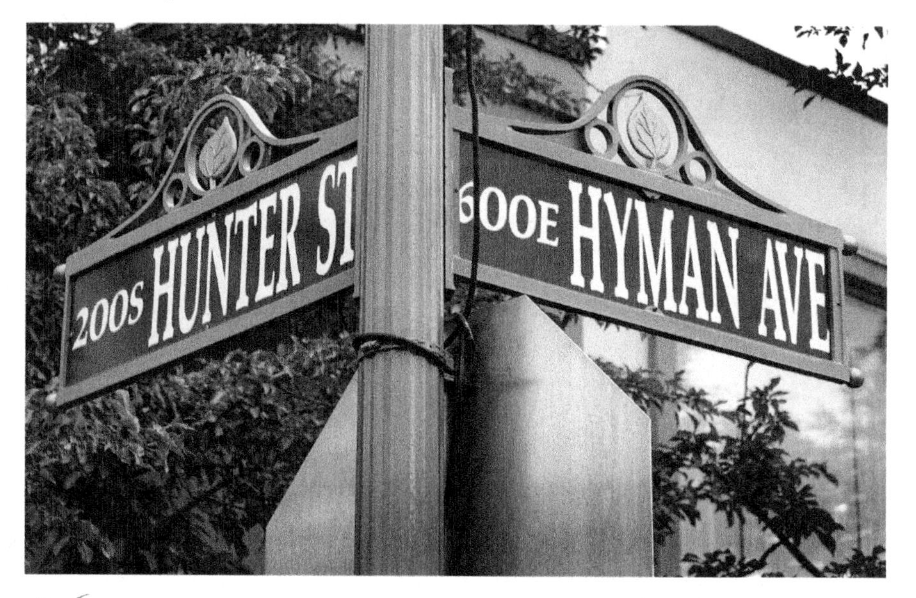

Here is a picture of the street sign. I'm sure I am not the only one who chuckles while driving through that intersection.

If your Granny Vagina Dilemma involves hunting for your elusive hymen gone astray, Aspen might be just the place to begin your journey. It could also be your solution.

Coming to Terms

Hymen—the thin, crescent-shaped membrane that partially covers the external vaginal opening.

Sign of a Virgin?

Some people think an intact hymen is a sure sign of virginity; however, many things can tear a hymen besides penetration during intercourse. Some examples are tampons, exercise, or pelvic exams.

Certain cultures place supreme importance on virginity at the time of marriage, often proved by bleeding with the first intercourse on the wedding night. It's not entirely out of the realm of possibility for the bride to undergo an examination ahead of the wedding, just to be sure her hymen is intact.

This chapter could read like a fairy tale, couldn't it?

Hymen Happily Ever After

Once upon a time there was a beautiful young maiden—only she wasn't technically a "maiden" any longer because, although she was old enough to know better, she had lost her virginity to an unscrupulous boyfriend. He told her that from the day he was born his family had promised him to the priesthood, and he just couldn't let his family's honor down; so he said, of course, he would be a priest. But before he took his vows to renounce the world and all its works and all its ways, he pleaded with the beautiful young maiden to have sex with him, which she had no intention of doing. Well, he argued how selfish she was to pass up one night of love just for the sake of holding on to her virginity when, after all, he was going off to a whole lifetime of celibacy (and other spurious arguments like that one).

So, she gave in, but soon regretted the error of her ways when she learned that the wannabe priest had lured all the other maidens in the village into bed with the same story.

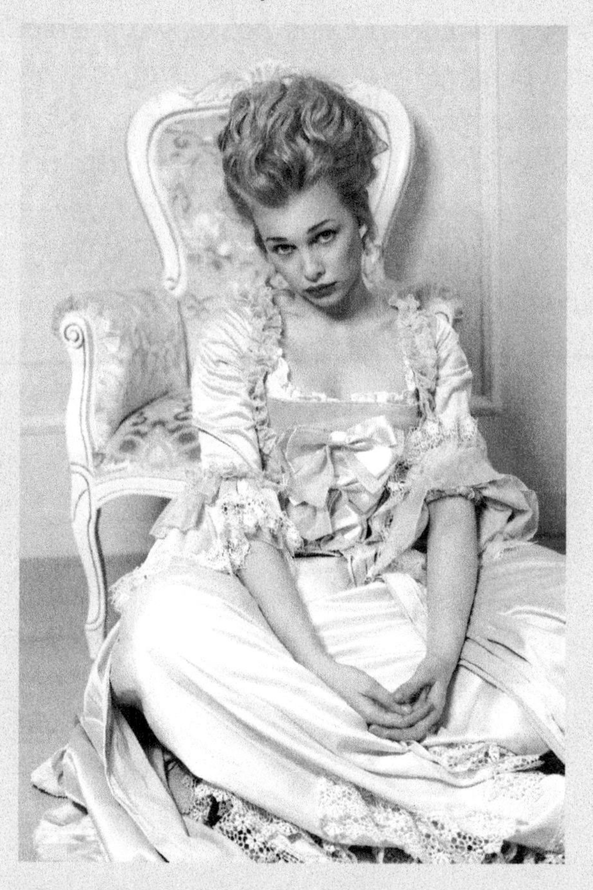

Bye and bye a handsome young prince from a faraway land rode into the village offering a fortune for a virgin bride, as his culture placed paramount value on a woman's virginity. He fell in love with our beautiful, young, no-longer-a-virgin maiden and made overtures toward her. This offer put her into a terrible quandary because, even though she was no longer a virgin, marrying this handsome prince looked like the only way for her to escape marrying the fat, pimply-faced butcher's son, who was her only other suitor.

The unfortunate girl ran to her fairy godmother and cried, "Oh Godmother, if only there were some way to confidentially regain my virginity that I so foolishly gave away to that rascal." Whereupon her fairy godmother, being not only a godmother but also a supreme gynecological surgeon, performed an emergency hymenoplasty (also known as hymen reconstruction surgery or hymen restoration). The torn edges of her hymen were put back together with the tiniest dissolvable stitches, which left no apparent scarring, so that even on inspection the delicate skin membrane once partially covering the opening to her vagina appeared intact once more.

Our beautiful young newly-restored maiden resumed non-strenuous activities in a few days, then coyly held the prince off for six to eight weeks while she healed, and on their wedding night her newly-restored membrane was ruptured with their first sexual intercourse. She bled a little, he was none the wiser, and they lived happily ever after.

It Can Happen to You

Fairy tales can come true; hymen restoration can happen to you, if that's what you desire. Whether tampon use, vigorous exercise, physical strain or sexual intercourse caused your hymen to rupture, laser hymenoplasty can repair your hymen, restoring it as if nothing ever occurred.

Although some women desire surgery because they want their hymen restored, more commonly I am called upon to correct congenital defects of the hymen. During your formation as an embryo, the hymen starts out as an obstructing membrane. A hole opens up, usually near the top of the membrane, leaving a crescent-shaped remnant at the bottom, which partially covers the opening to your vagina. If no hole develops at all, your menstrual blood will have no way to flow out of your vagina and can back up, causing serious problems.

If no hole opens up, serious problems may develop.

Frequently, the opening will not form completely, leaving a swiss-cheese type appearance or strands of tissue spanning over the gap. Patients whose hymen is completely closed or only partially open often endure menstrual pain, difficulty inserting tampons, and issues with sexual intercourse.

When a patient seeks hymen reconstruction, for whatever reason, I use delicate laser techniques to restore the proper anatomy.

A Note of Sensitivity

I do want to acknowledge and be sensitive to victims of rape or incest. Whatever reason you have for wanting or needing hymen surgery, be assured you will be treated with kindness, understanding, and respect.

That Covers It

Our third HUSH-HUSH chapter covered hymens, a subject women don't talk much about. (Well actually, there's not a great deal to say about your hymen, is there?) But next, we'll end the HUSH-HUSH section with a real page-turner, "Toying with Sex."

Chapter Nine

Toying with Sex

Your Sex Partner

A Gentle Reminder: In the context of our discussion, your "sex partner" is the person with whom you engage in sex. Gender of your sex partner is not the issue, nor is the type of relationship. Just for convenience, I'll refer to your sex partner as male.

Libido: A Very Important Topic

Here's a question about a very important topic: Why are women reluctant to talk about their ***libido*** (overall sexual drive) with their gynecologist?

I speculate that

- sex is taboo for women to enjoy;
- it is common for women not to have orgasms with vaginal sex; and
- women are embarrassed to bring up the subject.

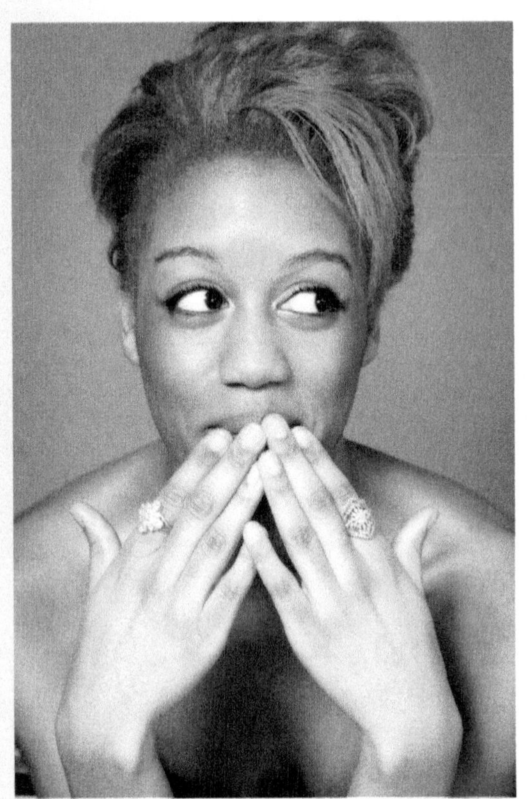

Bringing Sex Out in the Open

In my practice, I find it is rare for a patient to initiate a conversation about her sex life during our first visit. But over time, it is common for the topic to come up. I often ask about libido and sex as a routine part of an annual exam, during hormonal consults, or when evaluating pelvic organ prolapse.

As a rule, I'm the one who has to ask the question: "How is sex for you?"

"Oh fine," my patient might reply, when it isn't fine at all.

Or she might say, "It never occurred to me," indicating that the idea of how her sex life is going never crossed her mind.

Once I introduce the topic and we've established that it is safe to talk, my patients usually have plenty to say and the truth comes tumbling out.

Sex Life Dilemma: "My sex drive slipped a gear."

You might be surprised to know that decreased libido is common, especially as women approach menopause. I find my patients typically go through three stages of decreased libido:

Stage 1

"I'm fine once we get going, I just don't initiate sex."

Stage 2

"My husband thinks I don't love him anymore because I never seem to be in the mood."

Stage 3

"I couldn't care less if I ever have sex again."

Sex Life Dilemma: "Who needs sex, anyway?"

Although the complete physiology of female sexual response is outside the scope of this book, there are a few points that need to be addressed. Humans are sexual beings, and engaging in sex is normal behavior for us. When you tell me that you and your sex partner are no longer regularly engaging in sexual contact, I must ask how you *both* feel about that situation.

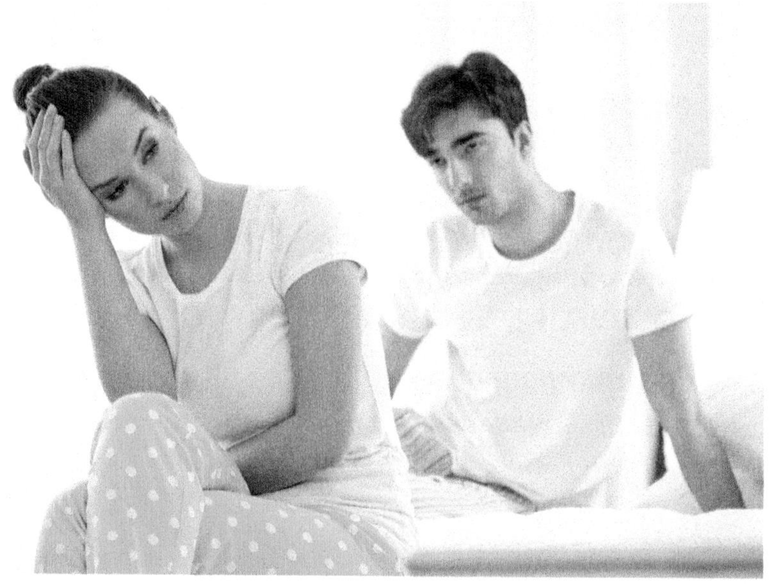

If the frequency and quality of your sex life is satisfying to both of you, then there is no problem; but Trouble in Paradise often begins when one of you isn't getting what you need out of your intimate relationship. Please don't try to fool yourself into believing that your sex partner is just fine without sex in your relationship. If sex is a problem for either of you, then it is a problem for both of you.

Underlying Causes

When your decreased libido becomes a problem in your sex life, you and I need to look for underlying causes:

- Anatomical issues—is your vagina stretched out or atrophic (dry, thin)?
- Are you on the birth control pill? Are you taking other medications that could interfere with libido? (Antidepressants are notorious for this side effect.)
- Prescription hormones—do you have enough of the hormones estrogen, progesterone, or testosterone? We can measure and replenish these hormones.
- Body image—if you're unhappy with your body image, you may lack self-esteem, leading to sexual dysfunction.
- Is your mind in the right place? Do you just need some time to relax first?
- Do you get the impression that you're only seen as "two boobs and a vagina?" (More non-sexual intimacy goes a long way with this problem.)
- Is withholding sex your passive aggressive way to let your sex partner know you are mad?

For Arousal a Woman Needs to Be

Anatomically normal;
Hormonally sound; and
Feeling good about her body image.

But Not

Too tired;
Too worried; or
Upset with her partner.

Usually, you and I will find one or more areas to work on to restore your libido. First, we'll strive to fix those anatomical issues and also to optimize hormonal imbalances (especially estradial and testosterone).

After you're in good physical health, I'll help you understand the libido and arousal response in women. We'll work on recognizing how difficult it is for you to respond when you are mad. Of course, when all is said and done, there is only so much that I can do to help you regain your lost libido, and sometimes therapy may be part of the answer for you.

Sometimes therapy may be part of the answer for you.

When You're Raring to Go

Now let's take a look at what happens after we have your libido perking right along. There you are—your vagina repaired and rejuvenated—you're ready and eager to start enjoying an active, satisfying sex life again. But wait! It may turn out that the sex life you're experiencing with your sex partner isn't all that satisfying to you.

Sex Life Dilemma: "I'm a sexy new woman—but my sex life is stale."

This Sex Life Dilemma presents itself in various ways:

"Wham-Bam – Thank You Ma'am"

Do you find your man sexually attractive, but he's just too fast to give you the pleasure you desire? Men are aroused visually, or even just by imagining sex. They think women's sexual arousal is just like theirs.

Men are the same the world over: they have their sex drive "ready at hand," youth to old age. Within a few minutes of starting intercourse, most men are finished with sex, while your orgasms are more

Men have their sex drive "ready at hand."

complicated. Often, you won't be sufficiently aroused for orgasm for another fifteen minutes or more.

A Penetrating Problem

Does he take it for granted that penetrating you during intercourse is the right way, and the only way, for you to experience orgasms? Then he doesn't know that, in order to be stimulated to orgasm, you do not require any penetration whatsoever, because most of your important sexual nerve endings are found on the surface of your vulva.

Boring Between the Sheets

Has your man become, to put it tactfully, "far less than sexy" in the bedroom? There could be an underlying reason he became sexually dysfunctional. Unfortunately, we don't have the time or space to explore this male topic, but erectile dysfunction is a problem of intense interest in the medical community today.

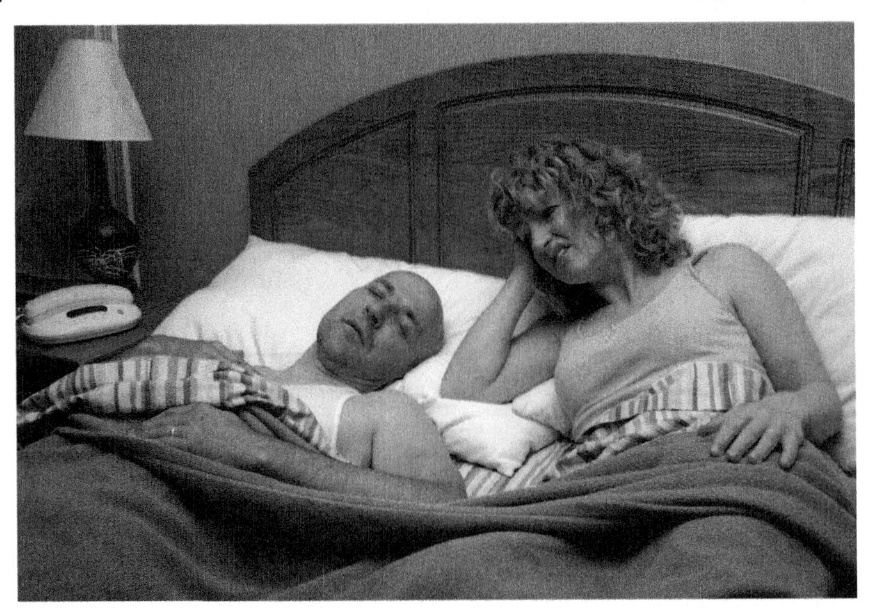

Perhaps your man simply might not be all that sexually attractive to you anymore. As men age, some let themselves become obese; or they stop paying attention to their personal hygiene.

Sex Life Dilemma: "So, what's a sex-starved woman to do?"

There's no reason for you to accept the idea that sexual pleasure will no longer be a part of your life. Today's women have heard the message: they have to take responsibility for their own sexual satisfaction. Here are some options:

Option One: Put It in Words

Even if he thinks he is the world's greatest lover, if you want your partner to give you real sexual satisfaction, you have to let him know what your needs are. One way to let him know is simple: Tell him.

You have to let him know what your needs are.

Option Two: Buy Him a Book and Read It with Him

Another tactic would be to surprise your partner with a good how-to book on sex. (What better present for Valentine's Day?) Try tucking it under his pillow. If he's the kind of man who's slow to take a hint, try putting it on top of his pillow—anything short of hitting him up 'side the head with it!

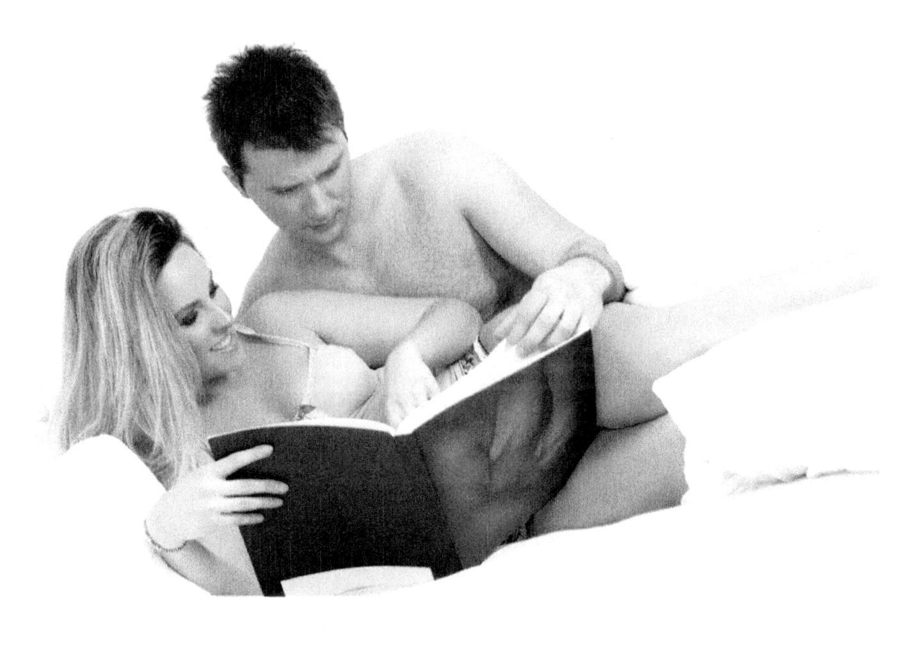

Books and More Books

On a recent trip to a leading bookstore, I discovered a whole shelf of sexually explicit (and I do mean explicit) books on every imaginable aspect of sex. Some were just downright shocking. Others, however, were written by credible authors who offered professional, practical, and useful information on achieving orgasms.

Option Three: Sex Toys Are a Good Idea

After I do pelvic repairs to restore and rejuvenate women's vaginal areas, I instruct them to abstain from sex for six weeks to let their new tissue completely heal. When my patients come back after six weeks for their check-up, I ask, "Do you have a dildo or a vibrator?" Half say yes. Half say no.

Do you have a dildo or a vibrator?

Start Out Easy after Vaginal Rejuvenation

The first penetration into your vagina after having it repaired often causes a sensation like being a virgin again because you are tight and tender inside. In the beginning, you have to go gently with that inner tissue. Perhaps it's time to buy yourself a present.

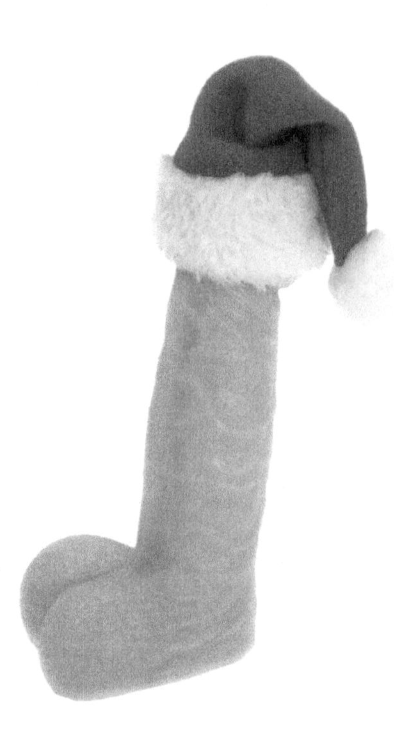

I might advise you to try using a vibrator before having sex again with your sex partner. This way, you will be in charge of how fast, slow, or deep it goes. Usually, after several times, your new vagina gets "broken in." After the reinitiation process, most women and their partners thank me.

Don't Put Away That Vibrator Just Yet

You are a sexy new woman. You want something you can be in charge of. A dildo can be a "girl's best friend" for pleasuring yourself and to augment the sexual pleasure you are (or are not) getting from your partner.

If you don't already own an adult sex aid, consider the fun of shopping for one with your sex partner. Perhaps you'll choose some exotic shape or texture. Or you might go for a no-frills style that doesn't make you feel threatened. It's best to find a dildo that is not-too-hard, not-too-soft, but firm and lifelike.

Shop Discreetly

If shopping for a dildo or vibrator in public sounds way too daunting, you can order one discreetly through my website: http://www.DrGailKing.com

Option Four: Throw a Sex Toy Party for You and Your Girlfriends

Now here's a way to empower yourself and others, and brighten up bedrooms all over town. Why go to the Adults Only Store when the store can come to you and your girlfriends in the privacy of your own home? Your friendly consultant (who obviously gave up all semblance of being embarrassed by these things) can demonstrate for you an array of adult novelties and products. There's lingerie to wear, lotions, creams, and sprays to put on. Then, from her suitcase of samples, she'll bring out a treasure trove of toys to titillate the entire pelvic region.

Add some food, perhaps champaign, and lots of sex talk. A sex toy party makes a Tupperware party pale in comparison.

Makes a Tupperware party pale in comparison.

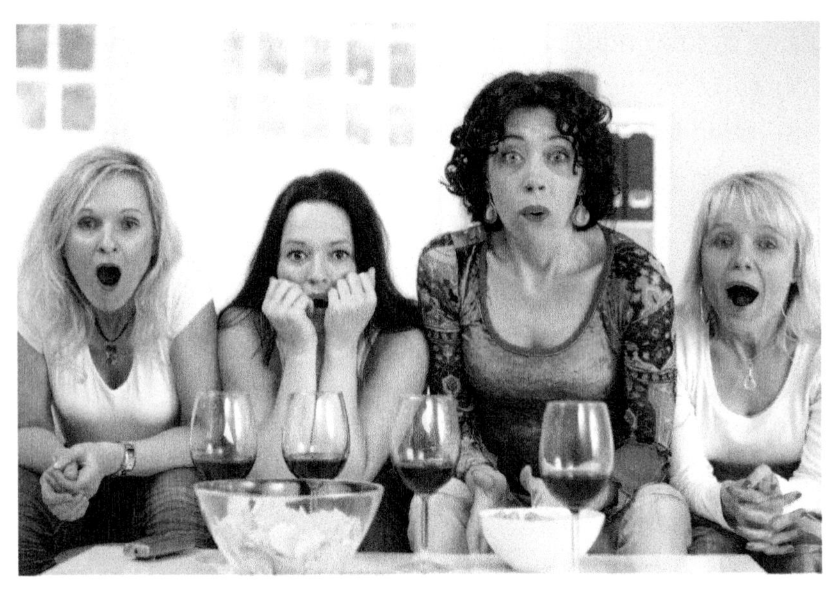

Option Five: If All Else Fails, Trade Him In for a New Model

Want to double your sexual responsiveness and boost your libido? You would probably notice a welcome change in your sex life if you were to change partners. New relationships feel exciting. It's sexually thrilling to meet someone new; your brain experiences the "in-love" effect all over again.

Seriously—Trade Him In? Probably Not

Obviously, for most women, changing partners isn't a plausible option. (But it was fun to think about, wasn't it?)

The Spark

Long-term relationships can lose their spark and become downright boring. Here's an interesting bit of scientific research regarding "loss of spark." ***Magnetic Resonance Imaging (MRI)*** *of the brain indicates that, usually over the course of two years in a relationship, a woman's brain actually shows a marked change in its response to thoughts of sex.*

The Brain in Love

In the beginning of a relationship, when a woman is "falling head over heels in love," MRI images indicate that a special location in her brain (the pleasure center) "lights up" with a response, even when she is only thinking about or seeing visual images of her new infatuation. (Interestingly, cocaine also triggers a response in this same area.) After about two years of togetherness, however, most women lose this intense response in their brain.

Researchers also found that couples who reported they were still madly in love, years into their relationship, continued to have responses in those same brain areas (much like couples who were newly in love).

End of the HUSH-HUSH Section

We have covered four chapters of personal topics that women discuss only in hushed tones. I trust you've garnered some good information. I also trust I've helped you overcome your fear of talking about sex with your gynecologist.

And now we're ready to move along to the next phase of a woman's life: "Part Four: Forever Feminine."

Part

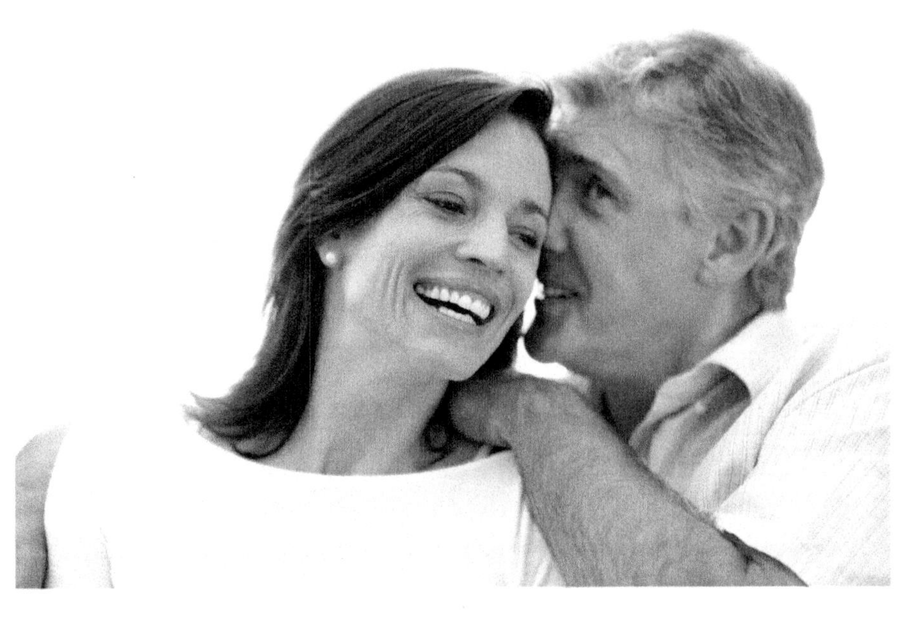

Four

Forever Feminine

Chapter Ten

Your Vagina in Menopause

Granny Vagina Dilemma: "Mother Nature ran off and left me behind."

So far, we have explored Granny Vagina Dilemmas arising when your younger vaginal muscles and tissue get stretched and weakened by childbirth and by other stresses and strains that life inflicts upon your lady-parts. There's one more Granny Vagina culprit hiding in the bush (no pun intended), and that culprit affects your vagina when menopause comes along, accompanied by a drop in the level of hormones produced by your ovaries.

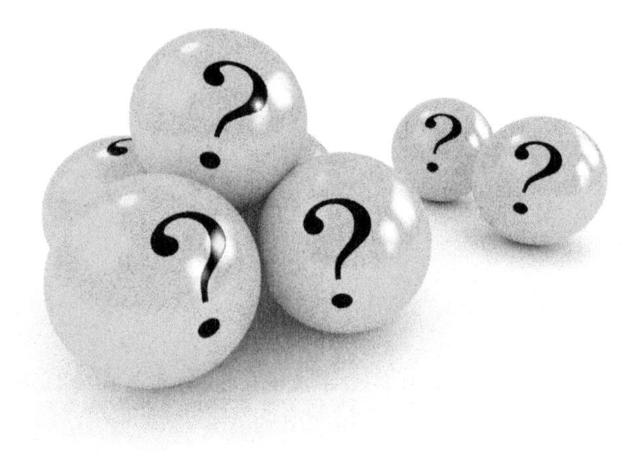

What about Those Hormones?

"Oh, yes," you say. "I have lots of questions about hormones and whether it's safe for me to take them." Well, hold on to those questions for just a little longer. In the chapter after this one, "Hormone Basics," we'll explore all that topic and more. But first, let's focus our attention on the changes your vagina undergoes around the time of menopause.

Raise Your Hand if ...

I am including this chapter for women whose Granny Vagina Dilemmas are attributable to lack of hormones. These readers are women whose bodies are no longer producing sufficient amounts of hormones (generally postmenopausal), and who are **not currently replacing those hormones** through hormonal (estrogen) therapy.

Coming to Terms

Menopause—your last menstruation is your menopause. We usually have to wait a year after your last bleeding to definitively say you've entered your menopause. The average age of menopause is around age fifty-two. For the rest of your life, you will be "***postmenopausal***."

Coming to Terms

Estrogen—a woman's defining natural female sex hormone, responsible for ovulation, menstrual periods and pregnancy. Estrogen also influences essential body functions.

The Big "M" and Your Vagina

Menopause is a shocker, no doubt about it. At the outset of menopause, changes within your ovaries cause the level of your most common hormones to drop dramatically. Menopause brings on a multitude of symptoms. It also leads to action in and around your vagina. Those vaginal changes are the focus of this chapter.

A Note about All Those Other Symptoms

Although I'm limiting my discussion of menopause to symptoms in the vaginal area, you'll find plenty of information available regarding all those other symptoms that menopause brings (like those infamous hot flashes, as well as weight gain and sleep problems). Menopause is one of the most written-about topics for women today. The shelves of your bookstore (or online bookseller) are well stocked with books on menopause. Search the Internet, and you'll probably conclude that every woman in the world who experienced menopause has something to add to the discussion.

An easy-to-read and practical book is The Menopause Makeover, The Ultimate Guide to Taking Control of Your Health and Beauty during Menopause, by Staness Jonekos with Wendy Klein, MD. The authors include information on pretty much every menopause symptom known to women.

Wasting Away

Granny Vagina Dilemma: "But I'm not eighty, how can my vagina look that old?"

It isn't a matter of age; it's a matter of ***atrophy***.

As estrogen levels in your body are depleted and not replenished, cells throughout your body lose their youthful vigor. One of the first areas where the effects can be seen is in and around your vagina.

When I examine a woman and see vaginal tissue that is no longer pink, soft, and moist, I tell her that her vagina looks old. Because it does look old. It has taken on the dreaded Granny Vagina appearance: thin, dry, gray.

Coming to Terms

Atrophy—withering or wasting away of tissue, organ or part of the body.

Step into My Office

Let me illustrate the progression of Granny Vagina Dilemmas caused by hormone imbalance—from least problematic to Disaster. Here are four examples compiled from patients I typically see. We'll start with this lady who doesn't think she has a problem. She is clueless about her condition because she isn't suffering any noticeable symptoms—yet.

Granny Vagina Dilemmas progress from least problematic to Disaster.

1. Stage of Denial: Postmenopausal/Not on Hormones/Not Sexually Active

Granny Vagina Dilemma: "Issues? Who, me? No, I don't have any issues."

First Postmenopausal Example: This patient actually has tissue changes due to decreasing hormones; however, she is not yet aware there's anything going on down there. She just went through her menopause. Because she is single and she isn't in a relationship or having sex, her only contact with her vagina may be when she takes a shower. She has not noticed outward signs of trouble.

This blissfully unaware woman is in my office for her annual exam. When I ask her if she is experiencing any problems, or if there are any issues she wants to discuss, she tells me, "No. No issues. None at all."

As I examine her pelvis, I can see that the tissue inside her vagina has lost its youthful pink appearance and has taken on an awful gray pallor. It is dry and has the potential to become dangerously thin: typical Granny Vagina.

When I see women patients with this condition, I first explain what I am seeing inside their vagina. Not surprisingly, they often find it hard to accept. A typical first response might be, "Well, it's not bothering me, so I see no need to do anything about it just now."

Further Risks

I then go on to explain that, unfortunately, there's more at stake here than just the appearance of the vagina. As tissue inside the vagina deteriorates, this condition opens the door to all sorts of potential risks. Some are common and treatable, such as the risk of vaginal infections or bladder infections. Other risks are more serious: thin, dried out tissue cannot hold the walls of the vagina firmly in place and other organs may begin to drop down into its space (all those prolapses we've discussed in previous chapters).

Use It or Lose It

A vagina without adequate estrogen, and one that is not regularly stretched from intercourse or with a dildo, will start to shrink and close up. I advise women to use a vibrator or dildo to at least try to keep their vagina from shrinking too much. It is truly a case of Use It or Lose It.

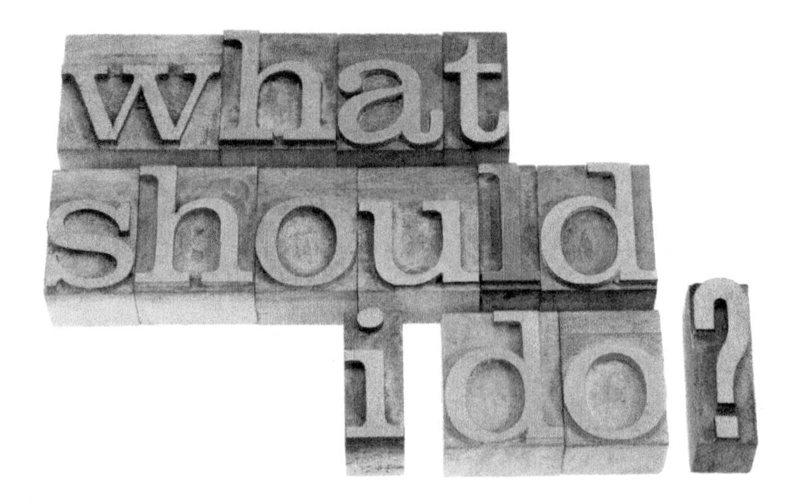

What Will This Patient Decide?

At this point in her visit, it's time for us to have the discussion about hormone replacement (lots more about that topic coming up in the next chapter).

Each woman must make a personal decision whether to start hormone replacement therapy. Some may not be willing to do anything, but will simply let their Granny Vagina go untreated.

Starting hormone replacement is a personal decision.

For the moment, let's leave this patient in our first example as she makes up her mind about hormone replacement, while we jump ahead about five years. Here we find a classic patient: one who is suddenly singing a different tune.

2. Classic Patient: Postmenopausal/Not on Hormones/New Sexual Relationship

Granny Vagina Dilemma: "Sex with my new boyfriend is torture!"

Second Postmenopausal Example: Here our classic patient is about fifty-seven years old. She has been postmenopausal for five years and during that time she was single and not in a relationship. After all those years of not having sex, she made a major life change: she began to date and recently entered into a sexual relationship with her new boyfriend.

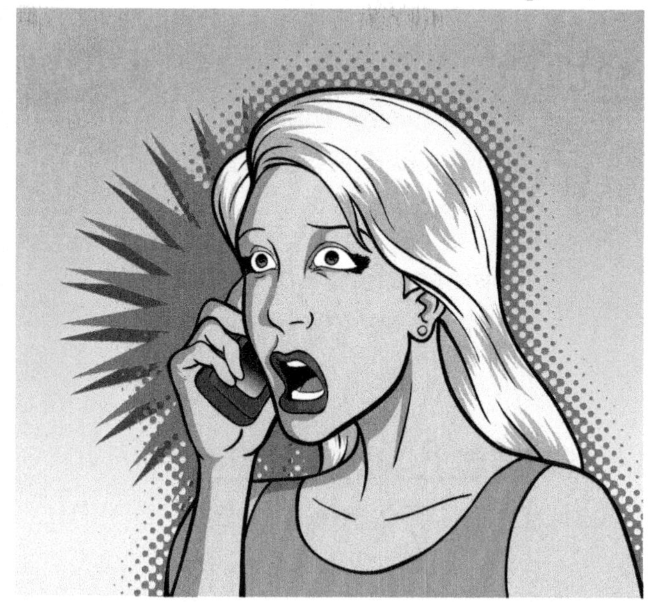

Soon I will get a frantic phone call: "Oh my God! We tried to have sex and it hurt. I was ripped, torn, bleeding. Now we have no sex at all."

For many postmenopausal women, painful sex in a new relationship is their call to action. They want their vaginal tissue to be soft and moist again.

During menopause, sex isn't as effortless as it was when you were younger because now the vagina lacks its lubrication and elasticity. Without estrogen, the vagina is no longer capable of readying itself for intercourse. As this patient found out, attempts at sex are painful, often followed by itching and burning. The vagina might also have shrunk; it is no longer large enough to accommodate a penis and is unable to stretch on its own.

What Can Be Done?

If there are no other signs of trouble except thin tissue vagina, I usually prescribe vaginal estrogen. But I remind these patients that their vagina didn't get this way overnight. When they begin treating their condition, it will take approximately six weeks of recovery time for their vagina to regain its healthy tone.

It may take six weeks for your vagina to regain its healthy tone.

If the internal dimensions and length of your vagina are severely diminished, we may need to employ vaginal dilation once the tissue is healthy enough to stretch again. ***Vaginal dilators*** are firm rubber inserts in sets that progress larger in diameter. They are used to gradually dilate or stretch the vagina back to a normal width and depth.

Next up is a postmenopausal woman who has been in a satisfactory sexual relationship for some time, but there's beginning to be Trouble in Paradise.

3. Trouble in Paradise: Postmenopausal/Not on Hormones/Continuing Sexual Relationship

Granny Vagina Dilemma: "I close my eyes, but I can't think of England."

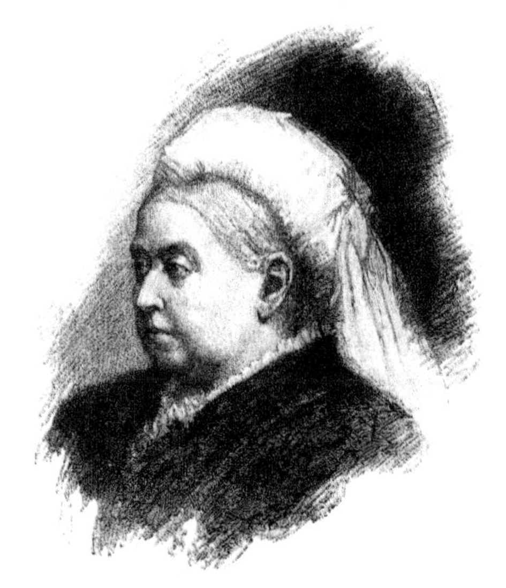

FORESTIER 1897

Victoria R I 1897

Although it might be an urban myth, historians allege that the popular saying Close your eyes and think of England is the advice given by straight-laced Queen Victoria to her daughter on the eve of her wedding. Sexual intercourse back in prudish nineteenth century England was thought of as a wife's duty-bound tolerance of her husband's aggravating sex acts.

Since Queen Victoria was known to love her husband dearly and they had nine children, it would seem she thought of England a great deal.

Third Postmenopausal Example: This patient is an older woman who currently is in a continuing sexual relationship—she has been married to the same man for years. They are starting to have marital problems: lack of estrogen makes it painful for her to have sex. Because she is having sex on an ongoing basis, at least her vaginal width has been maintained.

The woman in this example is obviously not enjoying sex because, simply stated, it hurts. When I examine her, I can see why. On the exterior, the fat pads surrounding her vulva have diminished. As her estrogen level dropped, collagen was depleted, leaving her external genital area saggy.

Looking into the interior of her vagina, I see those typical Granny Vagina symptoms: without estrogen the vaginal tissue is gray, dry, and lacking its normal folds. It is thin, like tissue paper. No wonder sex is painful.

Vagina with Estrogen:

- Interior is moist.
- Color is pink.
- Tissue is thick, elastic.
- Lining has folds (rugations).

Vagina without Estrogen:

- Interior is dry.
- Color tends to be gray.
- Tissue is thin, like tissue paper.
- Lining has no folds or elasticity.

Sex has clearly become a problem for this woman. Emotionally, her confidence as a sex partner is so far gone that she fears sex is simply no longer an option for her.

As this patient avoids sex more and more, issues begin to arise with her husband. She tells me, "My husband is concerned because he hurts me."

When women avoid or refuse sex, it's not unusual for men to think, "You don't love me anymore." They might not understand that she doesn't want sex because intercourse has become painful for her.

When women avoid sex, men often think, "You don't love me anymore."

Can This Marriage Be Saved?

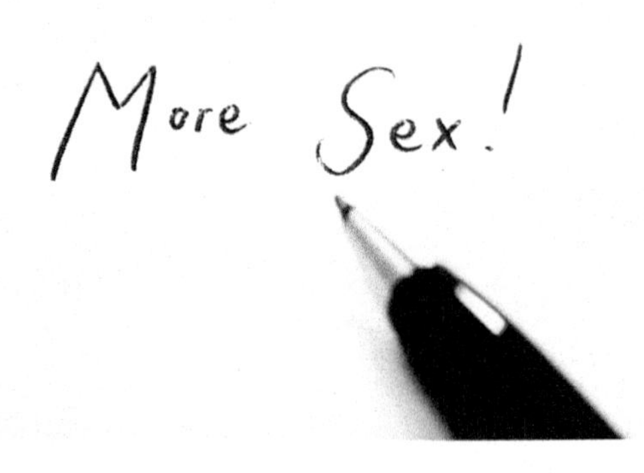

Don't be misled by foolish advice from well-meaning people who, obviously, are not experiencing excruciating pain when they try to engage in sex. If they were, they wouldn't say (and I quote directly from a recent article by a renowned sex therapist), "The cure: More sex."

More sex, indeed! How far would the patient in this example get by following that advice? For her, more sex would only equal more pain. She has a choice to make:

1. She can continue to do nothing about her painful condition, say nothing, and suffer sex in silence.
2. She can start avoiding sex with her husband, risking damage to her marriage.
3. She can begin treatment to remedy the source of her discomfort.

One choice for this patient may be to simply try using a vaginal lubricant with sex. There are many over-the-counter lubricants available. It is best to choose one that is water soluble, not one with a petroleum base like Vaseline.

This patient should consider hormone therapy. Hormone therapy can have a positive impact on your sex life, increasing your desire for sex and increasing your enjoyment when you have intercourse. Don't despair; once your hormone levels are restored, long-term relationships can still provide you with a satisfying sex life.

Other Potential Problems

Infections: Painful sex isn't the only problem postmenopausal women endure. Lack of estrogen after menopause changes the acid balance of the vagina, predisposing women to vaginal and bladder infections.

Prolapse: There can be problems even more serious than infections. Upon careful examination of patients without sufficient hormone levels, I'm likely to see signs of weakening in the vaginal wall that may already be allowing other organs (uterus, bladder, bowel, or intestines) to bulge down into the vagina. This bulging (prolapse) further impedes their ability to have sex without pain.

Possible Surgery Failure: Postmenopausal women in need of prolapse repair surgery face an additional challenge that younger women are not hampered by: it may not be possible to successfully put the prolapsed organ back in place. Once a lack of estrogen leaves vaginal tissue gray, thin, and dry, the tissue is not healthy enough to heal properly or to support itself after prolapse surgery. Stitches alone will not hold unhealthy vaginal tissue together.

After prolapse surgery, unhealthy tissue will not hold together.

The solution is to build up the vaginal tissue by providing the estrogen it lacks, commonly accomplished with the application of vaginal estrogen. There are several preparations that rejuvenate the vaginal tissue but are not absorbed by the bloodstream. Patients apply vaginal estrogen for six to eight weeks prior to prolapse repair. To maintain the repair, women need to remain on vaginal estrogen.

I'll give you more information about hormone replacement therapy, as a cream and all the other forms available, in the next chapter. But before we leave our postmenopausal examples, let me tell you about an older patient's Granny Vagina Disaster: the worst that can happen without hormones.

4. One Last Example: Postmenopausal/ Not on Hormones/Tissue Death

Granny Vagina Disaster: "It's yellow, it's yucky, and it's seeping out of my vagina."

Fourth Postmenopausal Example: Vaginal tissue that has been deprived of estrogen for a long, long time can actually start to "weep" fluid. Here, the cells have begun their death process. This atrophy distinguishes itself by a deep yellow, sometimes almost orange, discharge. Very scary. And very serious.

The cells have begun their death process.

I remember the first time I saw this type of discharge. I thought the patient might have a hole between her rectum or bowel and her vaginal canal. The fluid looked just like baby diarrhea. But there was no odor, and a culture did not grow any intestinal bacteria. Further testing proved that it was not cancer. The yellow yuck was seeping out from her vaginal wall.

To picture this disaster, think of an area of skin on your body that gets rubbed raw, like a "rug burn." Fluid seeps and oozes from a large denuded area that is usually covered by a vast layer of skin. The tissue surface inside the vagina is the "skin" of the vagina. And like skin elsewhere on your body, it serves as the protective barrier against outside elements such as bacteria.

This patient's oozing discharge indicated a total breakdown of her vaginal skin surface. Over-the-counter lubricants alone will not heal this type of discharge. The effective remedy would be estrogen.

How about Those Hormones?

As I noted in the beginning of this chapter, changes within your ovaries at the outset of menopause cause the level of your most common hormones to drop dramatically. That's why I have mentioned hormones frequently as I described your vagina in menopause.

Let's take a close look at those hormones in the next chapter, "Hormone Basics."

Chapter Eleven

Hormone Basics

Disclaimer

This book is not intended to provide a definitive discourse on hormones. For further information about the risks and benefits of hormone replacement, you'll have no trouble finding a tremendous amount of data that will help you make your own personal hormone decision. For example, I recently did an Internet search using the search term "hormone" and brought up 17,729 books.

Caution: Because research is rapidly accumulating new data on hormone therapy, be sure to check the publication date of information you find. On any given day you will find many books and articles hot off the press that describe the latest research findings. Authors of previously published information are (or should be) scrambling to update their material.

Window into Your Body

I'm including this chapter of basic information on hormones because hormones are extremely important. Deficiencies in hormones profoundly affect your health from head to toe. That's why, when I look at the condition of the tissue inside your vagina, it's like taking a peek into the window of your overall hormonal health.

Hormones are not the devil that they have often been portrayed in the media. Hormones are powerful chemical messengers that are secreted into the bloodstream, where they travel around and bind with appropriate receptors in the cell membranes of their target organs throughout the body. Once bound, hormones signal those cells to do something specific.

As nature intended, hormones are used by the body to function properly. Estrogen alone has nearly 2,000 jobs or effects on the human body.

Profound Impact of Hormones

Growth, Metabolism*—Hormones aid in metabolism, the efficient conversion of food into energy and other products your body needs to sustain life.*

Brain*—Hormones assist brain chemicals linked to thought processes; clarity and memory are targets for hormones.*

Collagen*—Without hormone replacement, older women may develop tissue-paper-thin skin (often seen on the back of their hands) from lack of collagen, a fibrous protein found in skin and other connective tissue.*

Bone Health*—Hormones control the bone-building process. You need to protect your bones from becoming fragile as you age.*

Organs, Muscles, Tissue*—Hormone receptors throughout your entire body and genital area enable organs and muscles to remain healthy.*

Vagina*—As we discovered in the last chapter, when natural hormones start to wane, deteriorating tissue in the vaginal area poses serious problems.*

Granny Vagina Dilemma: "Oh where, oh where, have my hormones gone?"

Natural changes in your female sex hormones typically begin around age forty. At that time, slowly and sporadically, the level of sex hormones working within your system decreases.

Coming to Terms

Menopause—the end of menstruation. The time in a woman's life when lack of natural hormones causes menstruation to cease, usually around age fifty-two.

Andropause—male menopause. The time in a man's life characterized by a slow and steady decrease in the amount of testosterone in the system, usually corresponding to the age of menopause in women.

Perimenopause—the time before actual menopause when natural hormone production begins to diminish.

Postmenopause—the time in a woman's life after her ovaries are no longer functional and she has stopped having menstrual periods.

Estrogen—a woman's defining natural female sex hormone, responsible for ovulation, menstrual periods and pregnancy. Estrogen also influences essential body functions. Women produce estrogen in their bodies in several forms:

(E_1) Estrone—the dominant form of estrogen in women after menopause, and in men.

(E_2) Estradiol—a form of hormone present in the ovaries and the dominant estrogen in the body prior to menopause.

(E_3) Estriol—the estrogen produced during pregnancy.

Coming to Terms cont'd

Progesterone—the natural female sex hormone that acts within the womb and placenta in connection with pregnancy (progestin is the version synthesized by drug companies).

Testosterone—a male steroid hormone produced in a man's testicles, also made in smaller quantities by women in ovaries and adrenal glands. Many doctors prescribe testosterone drugs to women. It is estimated that about one in five prescriptions for testosterone are intended for women.

Premarin, ***Provera***—names of non-bioidentical hormone products marketed by a leading drug company. The estrogen in Premarin originates with horse urine from pregnant mares (thus the name Pre-mar-in) and becomes one ingredient in a combination of estrogens. Provera is a non-bioidentical progestin.

Bioidentical hormones have a molecular structure identical to the natural female sex hormones that your body already makes (or more precisely, the hormones your body used to make before menopause).

The terms ***Bioidentical, Non-bioidentical, Synthetic, Natural, Pharmaceutical*** and ***Compounded*** will all be explained in greater detail as we move through this chapter.

Weighing the Risks and Benefits of Hormones

Some Women Say, "But I just want to age naturally."

Some women (usually women who are just approaching menopause and are not yet fully suffering its consequences) question the wisdom of interfering with the natural course of their body's aging process.

"Why interrupt or change something that nature has started?" they ask.

Think about what nature has started in your body: the body needs hormones to function properly, and without hormones, cells throughout the body have actually started the process of dying.

The body needs hormones to function properly.

Way back in our evolutionary past, nature never intended female human beings to live as long as we do now. For the first time in history, most women are living decades past their menopause. Although our mothers and grandmothers may have "aged naturally," along the way they had to suffer many problems due to lack of hormones. Today, women can choose not to decline that way.

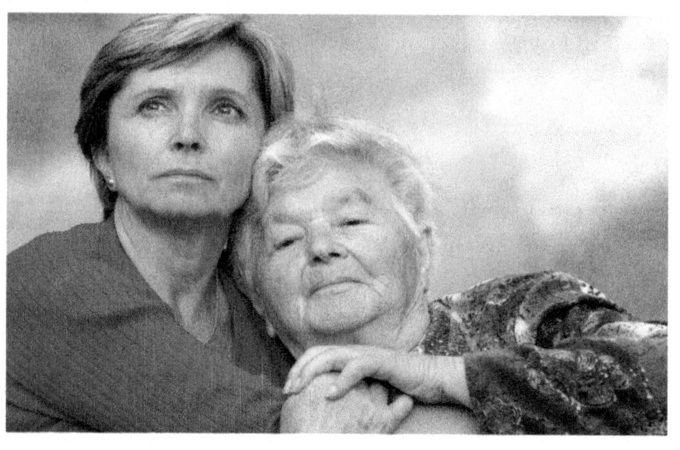

However, if you want to face your advancing years without hormone replacement, all the while enduring a host of problems throughout your body brought on by loss of hormones, that's certainly your choice to make.

A Common (But Ungrounded) Fear

Sometimes I hear a patient say, "I don't want to take hormones because I don't want to get breast cancer."

Women who voice this concern often think that, if they refrain from taking hormones, they won't ever get breast cancer. In this case, however, one thing does not necessarily lead to the other.

Cancer has many causes (for example, genetic mutations, toxic exposure, even viruses). Recent studies indicate that properly prescribed and monitored bioidentical hormones have not been shown to cause cancer.

Recent Studies

Cancer has many causes. Recent studies indicate that properly prescribed and monitored bioidentical hormones have not been shown to cause cancer.

Think about it. Why would hormones that your body produces abundantly before menopause suddenly turn toxic if they're replaced after menopause by hormones with an identical molecular structure?

So—Are Hormones Good or Bad?

There's not a definitive answer to that question because each woman has her own distinctive hormone challenge. Unfortunately, hormone replacement therapy has generated a good deal of confusion. When women go in search of relief from symptoms of menopause, they may find medical professionals who advise against the use of hormones and other medical professionals who are convinced that hormone replacement is beneficial.

Fortunately, times are changing—and changing fast. We now have more information than ever before. For instance, researchers have recently taken renewed interest in hormone replacements that are an exact copy of the body's own natural female sex hormones (bioidentical).

I provide my patients with the most accurate and up-to-date information about the benefits of hormones. Then I help them make an informed decision about whether to use hormone replacement therapy to alleviate their symptoms of hormone imbalance.

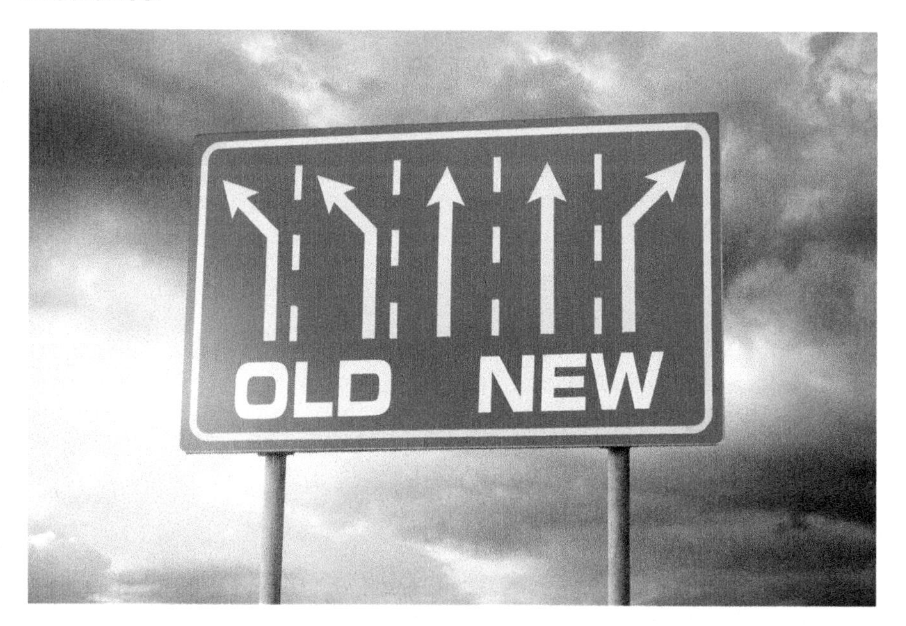

Beware Inaccurate Information

Remember the caution I inserted in my disclaimer above? You should be aware that researchers are rapidly accumulating current data on hormone therapy.

Much of what was published about hormones in the past ten years is likely to be alarmist and inaccurate in view of today's information.

Alarmist? Accuse the Government

You might wonder where those alarmist and inaccurate warnings against taking hormones originated. The answer: a government study. I've termed it the ***"Hormone Hoop-La."***

A Short History of the "Hormone Hoop-La"

Prior to 2002, postmenopausal hormone therapy was almost universally recommended to women. On July 9, 2002, however, after a quick interpretation, the conclusions of a controversial government study on heart disease, conducted by the Women's Health Initiative, were publicized. Part of the study was abruptly terminated and all women were warned to immediately stop taking all postmenopausal hormones.

Overnight, all hormone therapy for all women was demonized.

Millions of women panicked, terrified that their hormone pills would surely cause breast cancer and heart disease. They flushed their hormone pills down the toilet. Doctors stopped prescribing hormones for relief of menopause symptoms.

Looking back, it is clear that the study results, as publicized, were misleading.

Premarin®, or a combination of Premarin and Provera®, were the only hormones investigated. Premarin is high in estrogen from horse urine, a chemical form of estrogen that is not identical to natural female sex hormones produced within the human body. Provera is a non-bioidentical form of progestin. The biggest travesty is that the study report generalized the findings to all other forms of hormone therapy, as well.

Furthermore, the majority of the study's entire sample of women were already well past menopause when they were given the products to test. They had not been taking hormone replacements since their menopause (sometimes ten to twenty years earlier), and many already had underlying issues and increased risks.

The premise of the study was to investigate whether taking estrogen after menopause would decrease a woman's risk of developing heart disease; that is, it was a primary prevention trial.

How ironic is it that the women in the study were never tested to see if they had underlying heart disease before being enrolled in the study? Standard research protocol would demand that if you are trying to prove estrogen decreases the risk of heart disease, researchers must first be sure that heart disease is not present in the participants before the study begins.

The negative finding (that the estrogen tested did not decrease the risk of heart disease in the study group) was generalized to all hormone replacement therapy for *all postmenopausal women. A small increased risk of breast cancer was found in the group of women in the study who were given the combination of Premarin and Provera (the non-bioidentical Progestin).*

No increased risk of breast cancer was found in women using just Premarin. Positive findings of decreased colon cancer, decreased osteoporosis, and decreased risk of Alzheimer's disease were downplayed. In spite of the poor study design, the researchers declared that all postmenopausal hormone therapy should be restricted to use only for severe menopausal symptoms and only for a short time frame.

Now, after more than ten years of further analyzing the data, researchers have found many flaws regarding the study's design and the way in which results were interpreted and portrayed to the public.

For More Information

This summary was a short history of what I'm calling the "**Hormone Hoop-La**." An excellent in-depth analysis of the *Women's Health Initiative* study, as well as up-to-the-minute hormone information as it develops, can be found on the website http://www.hotflashhavoc.com.

New Findings

As newly emerging data is examined closely, some take-away points are now evident:

- There is a window of opportunity, around menopause, in which to initiate hormone replacement therapy that maximizes the long term health benefits.

- There are routes of administration that minimize potential risks.

Your Accurate Diagnosis

During your perimenopausal years (approaching menopause), your body shows subtle changes as it begins to lose optimal levels of female hormones. By the time of your menopause, these changes are usually accompanied by a range of uncomfortable and troublesome symptoms.

Whether you seek medical advice before menopause or after it arrives, accurate diagnosis of your condition is essential. In my office, I will do several things in order to decide whether to recommend hormone replacement treatment.

Accurate diagnosis of your condition is essential.

First, I will review your history and give you a thorough physical examination to evaluate your symptoms and overall health. With this information, I can determine if there are any other underlying health problems that might explain some or all of your symptoms.

If other explanations for your symptoms can be ruled out, the next step will be hormone testing. By measuring your hormone levels and the proportions of your sex hormones, I can determine your specific needs. Where hormones are indicated, I will make recommendations for the type of hormone replacement treatment that may be best for you, as well as the appropriate dosage.

Which Hormone Treatment

After we work together to diagnose your need for hormones, and assuming you decide to begin hormone replacement therapy, you might think that's all there is to it. Your decision has been made; now you can go home. Right? No, not so fast.

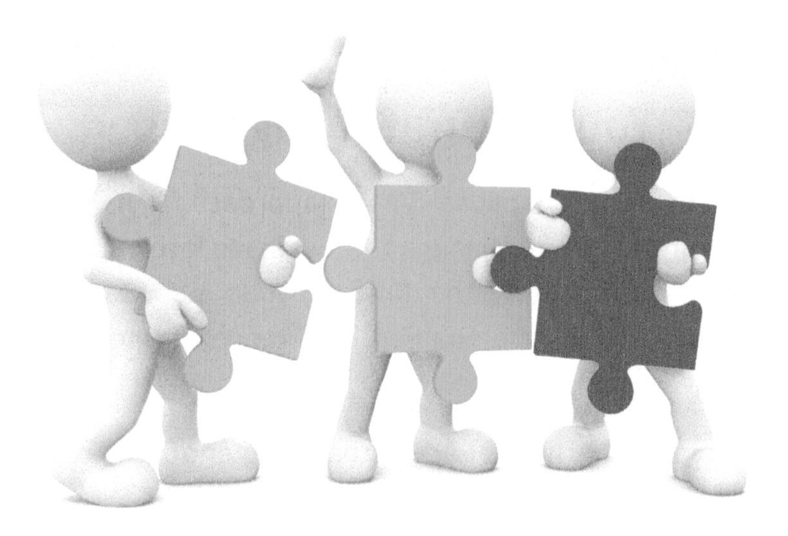

Three More Levels of Decision Making

There are a few more factors to consider and three more decisions to make:

1. First of all, we need to discuss the **forms of hormones** that are available.
2. Then, we'll determine **where you will obtain your hormones.**
3. And finally, we'll look at various **ways for your hormones to be administered**, and choose one that will work best for you.

Decision #1: Forms of Hormones

I like to start off by defining the medical terms for the different forms of hormones that are available (so that we will both be on the same page).

Bioidentical Hormones

Bioidentical means the hormones have a molecular structure identical to the natural female sex hormones that your body already makes (or more precisely, the hormones your body used to make before menopause). In your body, bioidentical hormones produce the same functional response as your own natural hormones.

> **Coming to Terms**
>
> ***Bioidentical*** refers to a substance with a molecular structure that is identical to a substance that the body naturally produces.

Hormones in bioidentical form have been in use since the 1930s. They only fell out of common use when a large pharmaceutical company began to market its own brand of non-bioidentical hormone replacement. Recently, there has been a resurgence of interest in the benefits of bioidentical hormones.

How They Work

Because bioidentical hormones have such close compatibility with your own natural chemistry, your body can metabolize and use bioidentical hormones as efficiently as your body's own natural hormones. Your body actually augments your natural hormone production with bioidentical hormones.

Your body augments natural hormones with bioidentical hormones.

How They're Made

To make a bioidentical version of a natural female sex hormone, chemists begin with material from sources found in nature (usually yams or soy). They extract a sterol from the cell membrane. From this sterol, bioidentical hormones

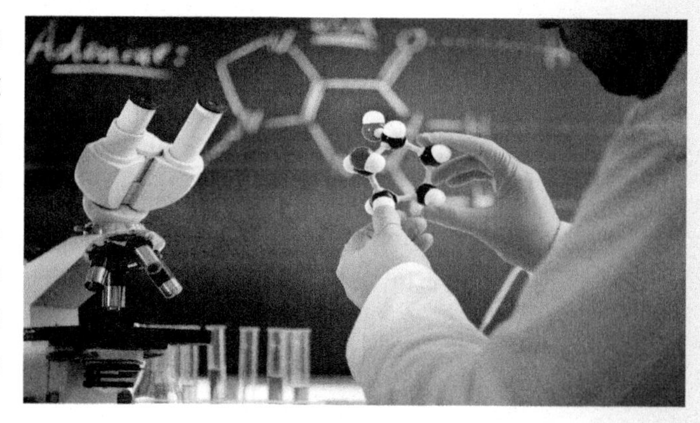

are synthesized that have the exact molecular structure of the body's own hormones—estrogen and progesterone.

Non-Bioidentical Hormones

Non-bioidentical hormones are sometimes referred to as "synthetic" hormones. Their chemical composition is not identical to those hormones produced by the human body.

Coming to Terms

Non-bioidentical refers to substances with a chemical composition that is not identical to those produced by the human body.

Is the issue "Synthetic?"

Non-bioidentical hormones are often referred to as "synthetic" hormones. Technically, however, even bioidentical hormones are "synthetic" because they must be synthesized (produced by a chemical process) from their original source, yams or soy.

Therefore, the term "synthetic" is not the issue; what's important is the chemical composition of the synthesized hormone you end up with—bioidentical or non-bioidentical—and how the human body recognizes that hormone.

What They Are

Non-bioidentical hormones are all other hormones that are not structurally the same as the natural female sex hormones produced by your body. Premarin, a leading brand of non-bioidentical hormone, originates with estrogen obtained from urine of pregnant mares, combined with other material to make a patented product. Non-bioidentical hormones also include birth control pills and brand names such as Provera and Norethindrone. Because they are not structurally the same as your body's own natural hormones, they may not produce the same functional response when they bind to your body's hormone receptors.

More Correct

Rather than saying, "I don't want synthetic hormones," it would be more correct to say, "I don't want non-bioidentical hormones."

Some Patients Tell Me, "I want natural hormones."

I prefer not to use the term "natural" because it can be misunderstood. For example, horse urine is very natural. It occurs naturally in every horse pasture in the world. The point is, hormones obtained from natural horse urine are not structurally the same as those hormones produced within your body. And some women do not want natural horse urine as their source of estrogen.

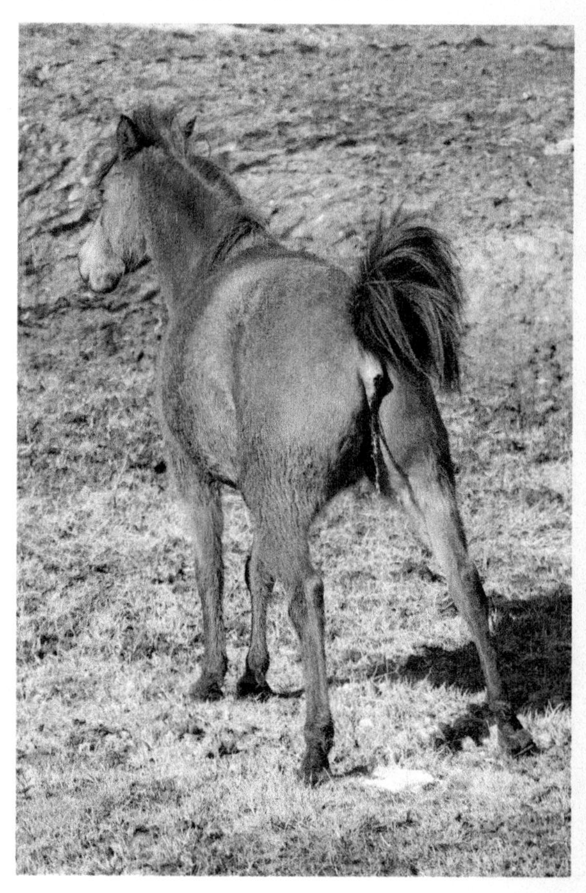

The only authentically natural human hormones (which would be very difficult to obtain) are those hormones produced inside authentically natural human bodies. Therefore, the only sources for natural human female sex hormones would be:

- Pregnant women's urine (which contains natural human hormones in minute quantities). Think how many pregnant women donors, peeing into bottles, it would take to supply the world's demand for hormones.
- A second source: human ovaries (but harvesting human ovaries would be considered cannibalism and certainly frowned upon ethically).

More Correct

Rather than saying, "I want natural hormones," it would be more correct to say, "I want bioidentical hormones."

Choosing the Form of Hormones for You

Based on the latest research, I prefer to prescribe only bioidentical hormones.

Ultimately, however, the choice is up to you. Each patient must decide for herself whether bioidentical hormones are best for her.

My Mother Is among the Dissenters

Of the many hundreds of women for whom I have prescribed bioidentical hormones, I have one patient who stubbornly holds out for non-bioidentical hormone replacement: that holdout is my mother.

Here is her true story—and, if you ask, she'll gladly tell it to you herself.

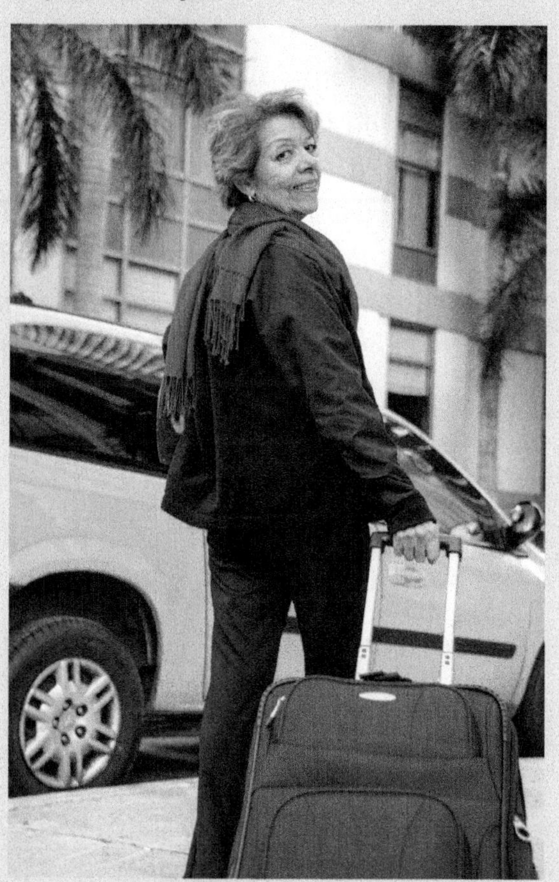

When Mom was thirty-four (way back in the 1970s), her ovaries were failing because of cysts. The medical wisdom of the day advised a hysterectomy and removal of the ovaries. The resulting drop in her body's hormones, however, suddenly brought on the worst symptoms of menopause all at once. Mom was miserable.

The doctor started my mother on Premarin (the hormone replacement regularly prescribed at that time), and her symptoms abated. She has taken that little purple Premarin pill faithfully every day since then.

When the Women's Health Initiative Great Hormone Scare hit the news in 2002, and women were advised to immediately stop taking all postmenopausal hormones, Mom studied the data that was made available and drew some conclusions of her own. She observed that the study's evidence showed a non-significant increase in breast cancer in women taking just Premarin. Because her female organs had already been removed, there was absolutely no chance for her to develop ovarian, cervical or uterine cancer. Furthermore, if she were to stop taking hormone replacement, those horrible menopause symptoms would return. Mom reasoned that, in her case, the benefits of hormone replacement outweighed the perceived risk.

Now, at age seventy-five, my mother still continues to take her non-bioidentical estrogen every day. At my suggestion, she tried switching to a bioidentical hormone, but said she "didn't feel as frisky" and preferred to stick with what has worked so well for more than forty years.

A recent pelvic exam showed that Mom's vaginal interior is moist and pink. Her tissue is thick and elastic with healthy little folds. Not at all a Granny Vagina.

Of course, over the years, my mother has had to contradict every doctor who questioned her continued use of hormones. But for her, this choice is simply a non-issue. Give up her estrogen? No way. It ain't gonna happen! (She jokes that she wants to have her hormone pills buried with her so that she can have them in the afterlife.)

Decision #2: Where to Obtain Your Hormones Pharmaceutical vs. Compounded

Pharmaceutical—Today non-bioidentical hormones and many bioidentical hormones are available pharmaceutically (meaning you can get your prescription for them filled at your local pharmacy).

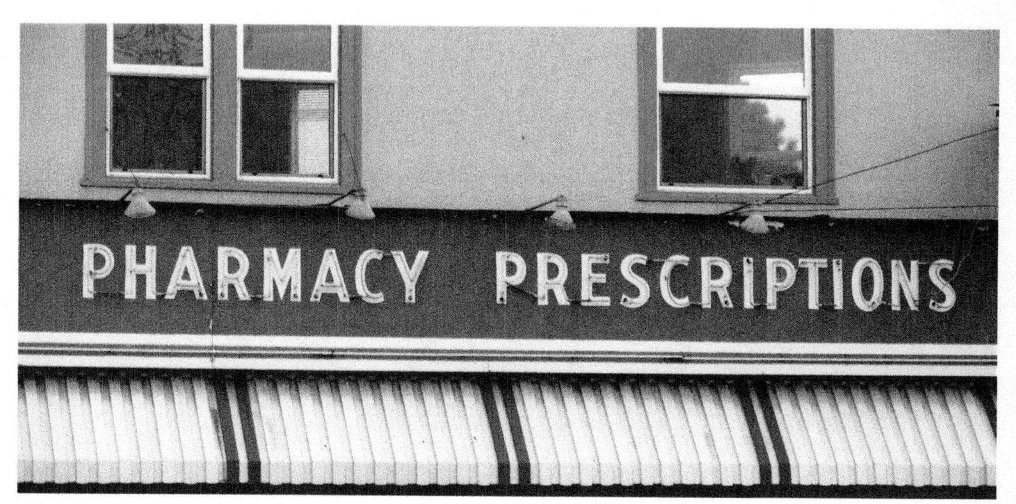

They are produced and marketed by major drug companies and come in many forms. Some are available as generic brands, which are less expensive than brand-name products. Prescriptions for many pharmaceutical hormones are covered by insurance.

Compounded—Hormones that are made to order for each patient must be compounded. They are available only through specialized compounding pharmacies that take bioidentical hormones and combine them into individualized formulas designed to meet each patient's singular needs. If your hormone treatment includes a compounded product, we will choose a reputable compounding pharmacy to fill your prescription. You need to be aware of the cost involved in using bioidentical hormones that are individually formulated; also, insurance does not generally cover compounded prescriptions.

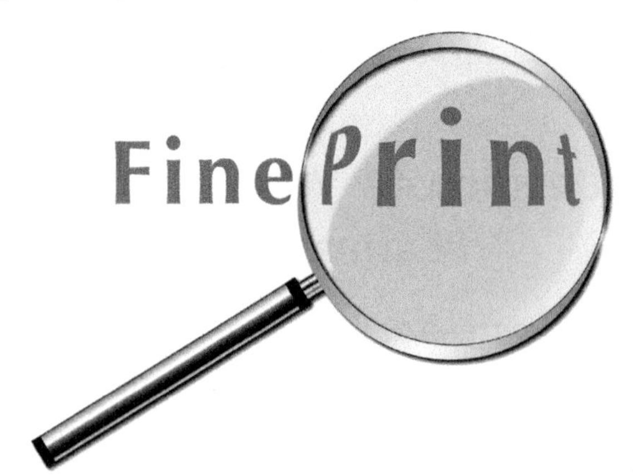

Insurance—Read the Fine Print

Health insurance generally covers hormones that you can get with a prescription at your local pharmacy.

Health insurance does not generally cover made-to-order hormones that you get with a prescription at a compounding pharmacy.

Which Type of Hormone Is Best—Pharmaceutical or Compounded?

Some doctors recommend only using hormones that are manufactured by pharmaceutical companies and available by prescription from your local pharmacy.

Other doctors recommend only using hormones that are compounded specifically for each patient's individual needs and only available by prescription from compounding pharmacies.

In my practice, I do not limit my patients to one or the other because each patient's needs are unique to her alone. Sometimes a "ready-made" pharmaceutical hormone formula may be the right one for a patient. Another patient may require a hormone formula that can only be obtained from a compounding pharmacy.

Decision #3: How Should Your Hormone Therapy Be Administered?

The ideal hormone therapy is effective and tolerated by your body.

Today you will find a wide range of hormone preparations to choose from. Each delivers the necessary hormones to your body in a different way. There are many factors to consider:

How Long Will You Be on Hormone Replacement?

When deciding whether you want a pill, a patch or something else, you should ask, "How long do I have to stay on hormone replacement?" The answer is: for as long as you want the benefits to last. In most cases, you should consider this therapy a long-term decision.

How Long Must the Repair Last?

If you had vaginal tissue repaired, you will need to stay on hormones to keep your tissue healthy enough for the repair to stay intact. How long do you want this repair to last? Your lifetime? Do the math.

Is It for Vaginal Dryness?

Estrogen replacements applied directly inside your vagina are very effective in helping restore moisture, thickness, and elasticity to dry, atrophic vaginal tissue. They can relieve irritation, itching, and burning caused by loss of your natural hormone, estrogen. Your vagina will be lubricated and the blood supply in the area replenished, enhancing sexual arousal.

You can refer back to Estrogen Therapy in chapter four, "What's a Woman to Do?" for our discussion of vaginal estrogen options—vaginal tablets, rings, creams, suppositories.

How Will Your Body Absorb Each Form?

Some estrogen replacements are absorbed systemically. Applied topically as a hormone-enriched formula, the estrogen gets absorbed rapidly into your bloodstream and lymphatic system. Taken in pill form, however, only a portion of a dose actually reaches estrogen-sensitive tissue because it must pass through your liver, where liver enzymes change some of the estrogen. Thus, oral estrogen doses need to be larger than topical doses.

Oral estrogen doses need to be larger than topical doses.

Is This Form Convenient to Use?

Think about whether you will be able to use the chosen form consistently and correctly. You know yourself. How well would you do with a messy hormone cream you had to apply twice a day, every day? You might prefer the convenience of a hormone patch that you change one or two times per week, or a vaginal ring that only needs to be replaced every three months.

What Is the Dose?

Using a patch, for instance, you can take a lower dose than with a pill because hormones from a patch on your skin are absorbed directly into the bloodstream. Pills taken orally get metabolized through the liver before reaching the rest of your body.

Choices for Administering Hormones

Pills and capsules that you swallow
Sub-lingual tablets (under the tongue)
Sub-dermal pellets (under the skin)
Intra-vaginal rings
Intra-uterine devices
Patches
Creams
Gels
Suppositories
Sprays

Importance of Monitoring

No matter which form you choose—hormones available at your local pharmacy or hormones compounded just for you—it is imperative for your hormone use to be closely monitored over time. Your general health, as well as your hormone level, needs to be professionally observed throughout your period of hormone replacement therapy.

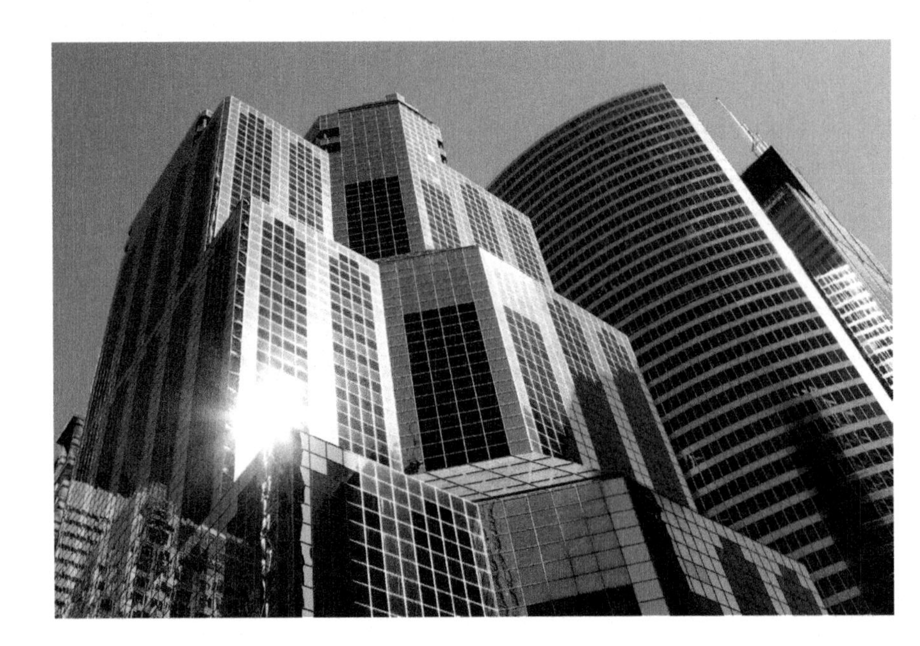

A Note about Big Pharma

In America, we tend to be quick to criticize large pharmaceutical companies (Big Pharma) for their role in development of new drugs. But let's step back and look at what has transpired in the field of hormone products since the Great Hormone Scare (Women's Health Initiative study) of 2002.

Until recently, large pharmaceutical companies predominantly manufactured and sold their proprietary formula of non-bioidentical hormones. Why? This form was the type of hormone replacement that doctors generally prescribed (when and if they prescribed hormones at all).

In the years following 2002, new information emerged regarding the benefits of hormone therapy using bioidentical hormones with a structure identical to the natural female sex hormones in your body. Masses of women began demanding bioidentical hormones for relief of their postmenopausal woes. In response, this demand for bioidentical hormones was met largely by independent compounding pharmacies that use naturally occurring substances to synthesize bioidentical hormone preparations.

Before long, Big Pharma recognized the market opportunity in offering bioidentical hormone preparations. In order to turn a profit, however, these pharmaceutical companies needed patentable products. Naturally occurring substances, such as yams and soy, cannot be patented.

The patent process is integral to the American marketplace. The government grants patents on new, innovative products. However, research and development of new pharmaceutical products requires a huge investment. With a patent, a company can manufacture a new pharmaceutical product exclusively for a period of time, without competition, in order to recoup their monetary investment in developing it. Because of patent protection, many new products are developed and made available to all of us.

Because pharmaceutical companies cannot patent naturally occurring bioidentical hormone substances, they have begun to patent their own original delivery system for these hormones: for example, bioidentical hormones imbedded in a specially designed patch, cream, or spray. Many of these patented products are becoming available with a prescription at your local pharmacy.

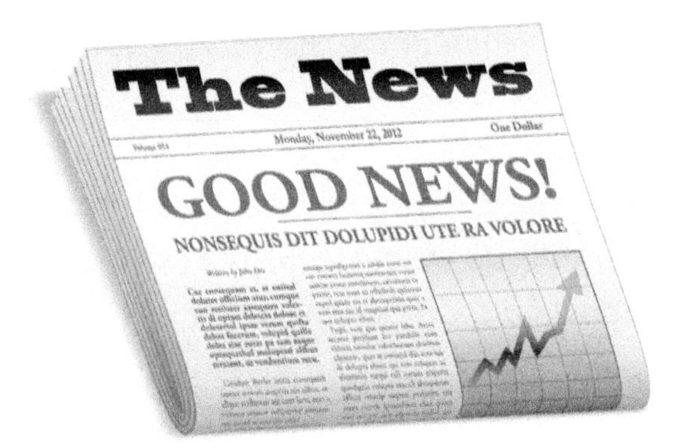

The Good News

All this activity means good news for us: we now have more bioidentical hormone choices.

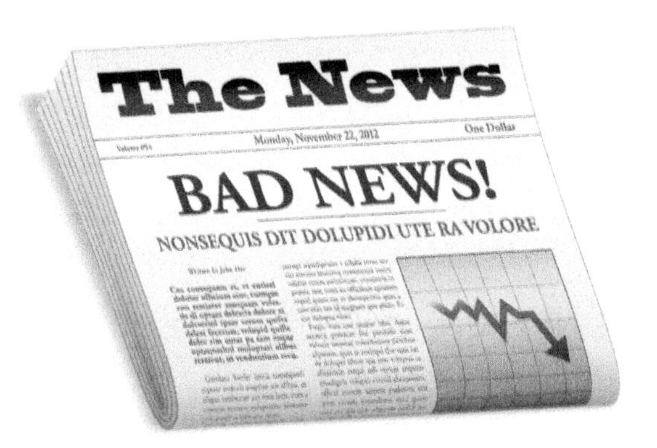

But Is There Bad News?

I heard that there is an effort, currently spearheaded by some large pharmaceutical companies, to have independent compounding pharmacies outlawed in order to eliminate competition to Big Pharma.

Without compounding pharmacies, however:

- Hormones and individualized drugs would not be available in combinations other than those commercially available at traditional pharmacies.
- Patients could not obtain non-standard doses or different routes of delivery, when necessary.

- Drugs or hormones that are not commercially manufactured by large pharmaceutical companies would disappear from the market.

Time to Move On

I trust you have learned valuable information from reading these two chapters. Now you know that you can achieve hormonal balance, bringing out the best in you in each transitional period of your life.

I want to conclude with three great chapters that will complete your makeover into a Savvy Woman. We'll discuss vaginal virus, your annual exam, and that question you asked way back at the beginning of the book, "Why didn't anyone ever tell me?"

Part

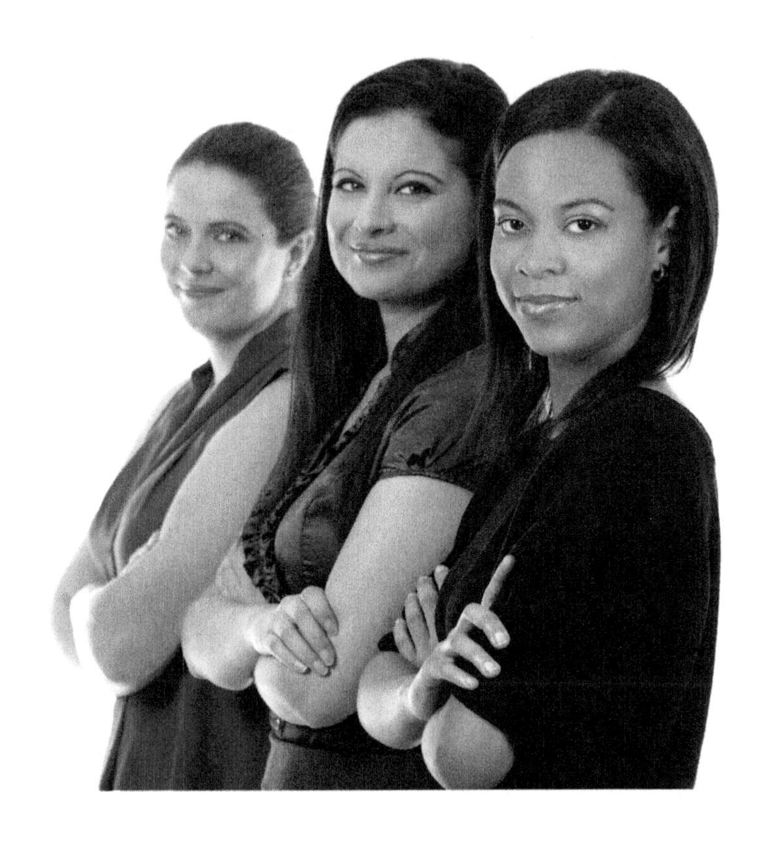

Five

The Savvy Woman

Chapter Twelve

You've Gone Viral

Note: In this chapter, I discuss three important issues in the same language I use when explaining them to my patients. I intend the information to be a resource; readers seeking medical advice should consult with their own physician.

You're on Your Way to Becoming a Savvy Woman

Throughout this book, you've been armed with lots of useful information to help you avoid the dreaded Granny Vagina. Now it's time to consider what it will take to keep your vagina perky and functioning well—the way Mother Nature intended.

After all, every woman wants to be sure all her lady-parts are healthy:

- Nothing falling out
- Not infected
- Not leaking

- Not obstructed
- Not painful
- No vaginal irritation
- No yeast infections

What better place to start than by scheduling regular check-ups with your healthcare professional. In your annual exam, any Granny Vagina Dilemmas can be identified and headed off at the pass. At the same time, screening tests can check for abnormal cells on your cervix, which could turn into cancer over time.

You know the old saying: An ounce of prevention is worth a pound of cure.

Screening Tests

In this chapter we will take an in-depth look at screening tests and the role of viruses in cervical cancer.

Viral Vagina Dilemma: "I don't feel bad, so why do I have to get screened?"

Because cervical cancer often does not cause symptoms until it reaches an advanced stage, it is important to get screened even when you seem to be healthy. Your cervical cancer screening may include both a Pap test and HPV testing.

Pap Test

Your Pap test checks for abnormal cells on your cervix. We use the Pap test to help us identify problems that can be found and treated before they ever turn into cancer. During your annual exam, I'll take a sample of cells from your cervix and send it to a pathology laboratory to be analyzed.

HPV Test

I may request the pathology laboratory to test for ***human papilloma virus*** (HPV) at the same time it analyses your Pap test. HPV is a common virus that infects skin cells, and some HPV strains can cause cervical cancer.

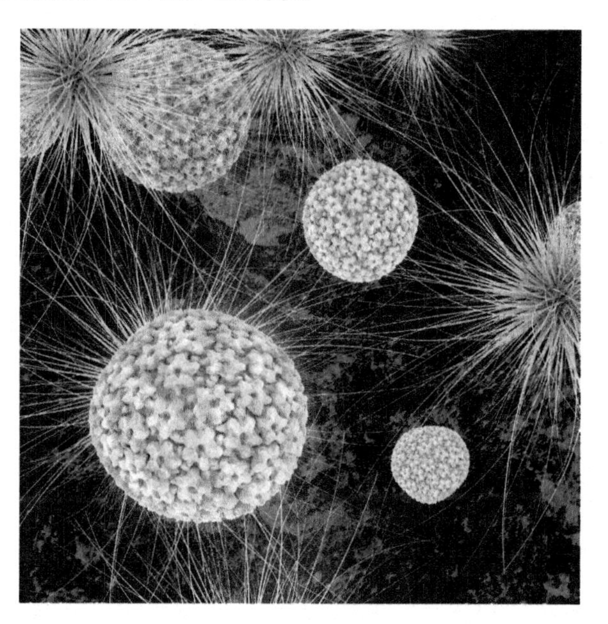

HPV is not HIV

HPV is not the same as HIV (the AIDS virus), nor is it the same as the herpes virus. All these viruses can be passed on during sex, but they do not cause the same symptoms or health problems.

Going Viral

Viruses Cause Cancer?

Some viruses do. Certain HPV types are responsible for changes that can lead to cervical cancer over time by causing normal cells on your cervix to turn abnormal. These abnormal cells can turn into cancer if they are not found and treated by your doctor.

Coming to Terms

Abnormal cells are sometimes called ***precancer*** because they are not normal, but they are not yet cancer.

To date, researchers have identified more than one hundred fifty HPV viral types. We use numbers (1-150) to distinguish one type or strain from another. Not all these strains have the potential to induce precancerous and cancerous growth. The ones that do have this potential are referred to as "***High-Risk Human Papilloma Virus***" (or HRHPV). There are approximately fifteen high-risk HPV strains.

The Villains: HRHPV

The HPV strains that have the potential to induce precancerous and cancerous growth changes are referred to as "High-Risk Human Papilloma Virus" (HRHPV).

Viral Vagina Dilemma: "I'll just be careful and avoid catching HPV."

That's not impossible, but in our society HPV would be awfully hard to avoid. The human papilloma virus is highly contagious. This virus is a sexually transmitted infection, transmitted by means of direct contact with another infected person. It is estimated that eighty percent of the population carries HPV, (and we just might not be smart enough to figure it out in the other twenty percent). Most of us become exposed during our first few sexual encounters.

Remember, your risk of contracting HPV, or other sexually transmitted infections and diseases, isn't limited to your current sexual partner. You are also exposed to every other person your partner ever slept with ... and anyone else that other person ever slept with ... and so on ... and so on ...

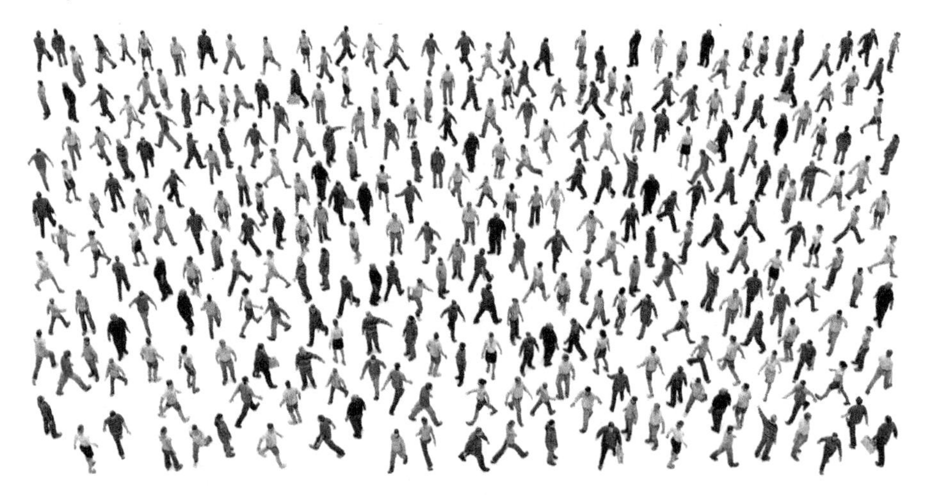

Viral Vagina Dilemma: "Can't I 'clear' the virus, or just wait for it to go away?"

Nope. Once you contract HPV, your body does not eradicate it. If we say someone has "cleared" the virus, that statement doesn't mean the virus went away. With most young, healthy individuals, we say they "clear" the virus when their immune system kicks in and makes the virus go dormant. This pesky virus will still be there—but not actively growing and dividing—just waiting its chance for your immune system to weaken so that it can invade your tissue and start growing again.

Once you contract HPV, your body does not eradicate it.

High-risk HPV may start growing when your immune system becomes weak. Then, after a period of time, the virus usually goes dormant again. Any condition that further weakens your immune system increases the chance the virus will start growing once more, and it will continue actively growing for longer periods of time. The length of time the virus remains actively growing

High-risk HPV may start growing when your immune system becomes weak.

(not dormant) determines the time you are at the most risk for development of cancer.

Viral Vagina Dilemma: "What If I've not had sex in years. How long might it take for cancer to develop?"

While it is dormant, high-risk HPV does not have the capability of causing cancerous growth. But anytime your immune system becomes weak enough to allow strains of high-risk HPV to infect your tissue, the virus turns on genes in your cells that induce growth. These genes usually have checks and balances, preventing runaway, unregulated growth; but high-risk HPV circumvents those checks and balances. The longer the virus actively grows, the more likely it is that your infected tissue will become cancerous.

The average time from initiation of viral growth to the stage that is one step away from cancer (***carcinoma in situ***) is two and a half years. Sometimes change happens much faster. I have personally seen women with no sign of precancerous changes on their cervix one year and carcinoma *in situ* the very next year.

Viral Vagina Dilemma: "Is it just cervical cancer I need to worry about with HPV?"

No, that's not all. Medical science implicates HPV in many more cancers, not just cervical cancer. Vulvar skin-type cancers (on your external genitalia) and vaginal cancer (in your vaginal canal) are caused by high-risk HPV. That's why you may still need to be screened for precancerous changes even after a hysterectomy.

Medical science implicates HPV in many cancers.

In men and women alike, some cases of anal cancer and also oral cancer are now recognized as being associated with high-risk HPV infection. Typically, doctors screen for anal cancer during a colonoscopy exam. As of now, however, there is no screening test available for high-risk HPV oral cancers. Most of the time, doctors find oral cancer in an advanced stage once it spreads to lymph nodes in the neck.

Viral Vagina Dilemma: "Hooray! My HPV screening test came back 'negative.'"

Don't celebrate just yet. A negative result could mean you do not have a type of HPV linked to cervical cancer. Or it could mean you have contracted the high-risk HPV virus, but it is currently dormant.

Here's how I explain dormant viruses to my patients: HPV is much like other common viruses. Varicella zoster virus is sneaky. If you contract this virus as a child, you develop chickenpox. After your initial episode of chickenpox resolves, you may be left with a few slight scars on your skin. But inside you, in certain nerve cell bodies, varicella zoster virus remains dormant without causing any symptoms. After many years, the virus can become active again in these nerves, triggering the painful, blistering skin rash we know as shingles.

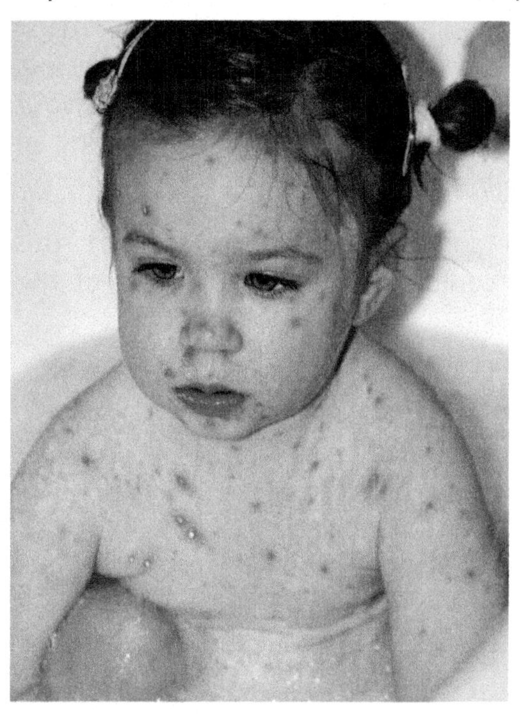

Also think about the herpes simplex virus. Once you've contracted this one, it's going to be with you forever. Now and then it will flare up and you might break out in cold sores or fever blisters, but this flare-up won't happen every day. Soon after a breakout, herpes simplex virus goes dormant, waiting to pop up again just when a cold sore is the last thing you want to have erupting on your lower lip.

Viral Vagina Dilemma: "OMG! My HPV screening test came back 'positive.'"

What should you do if your HPV screening test comes back with positive results?

1. Don't panic. You are not alone. Researchers estimate that eighty percent of the population carries HPV.
2. Get your cancer screening tests at regular intervals that will be determined by you and your doctor, based on your personal risk factors.
3. Keep yourself and your immune system healthy. Stress weakens your immune defenses (so calm down). Certain foods and supplements have been shown to boost your immune system. Look around and you'll find a wealth of information on this subject.
4. We don't yet have conclusive data to support this suggestion, but you could consider getting one of the current vaccines.

Vaccines? Did You Say Vaccines?

FDA-Approved Guidelines

The Food and Drug Administration (FDA) has approved two brands of HPV vaccine, and these are available on the market (Gardasil and Cervarix). Both vaccines protect against certain strains of high-risk HPV, if you've not yet been exposed to those strains. The FDA has not approved either of these vaccines for treating existing HPV or cervical cell changes.

The vaccines are recommended for girls and boys starting as early as age nine, because vaccination is most effective when given before a person's first sexual contact.

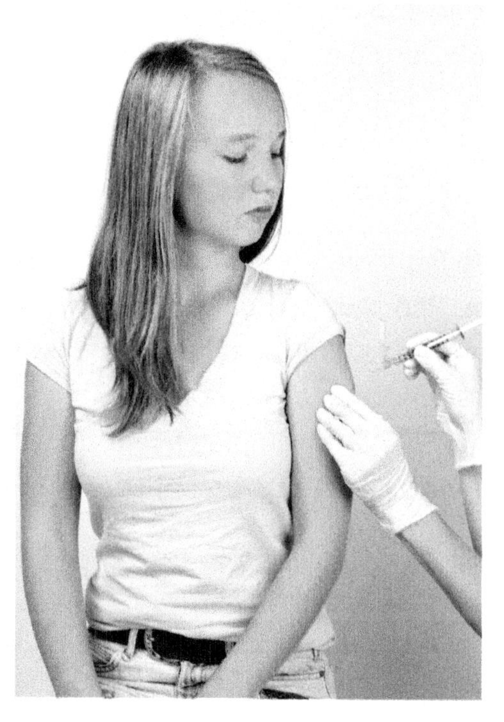

Vaccines Prescribed "Off Label"

Gardasil and Cervarix may one day become available to women in other age categories if these vaccines are found to be safe and effective for them. In the meantime, I have prescribed these vaccines "off label" for some of my patients.

Off-Label Prescribing

*The FDA approves new medications and vaccines for certain indications. This approval means the manufacturer did studies proving their product was effective for a specific condition. Once a manufacturer makes a medication available on the market, physicians may also prescribe it for other conditions or in circumstances that the FDA did not specifically say was an indication. The term for such prescribing is "**off-label**" use. Common examples would be prescribing some birth control pills to help with acne, or Viagra for use in female arousal disorder, not just for male erectile dysfunction. In these instances, the doctor informs the patient that the medication being prescribed has not been approved by the FDA for this use.*

Moving Right Along

I have explained your HPV screening test first, so that you will understand the role high-risk HPV plays in development of cervical cancer. Now we're ready to move along to your other screening test—the Pap test.

Your Pap Test

Most of you are familiar with the Pap test; it's one of the easiest tests you'll ever have done. The Pap test is usually not painful but might be a tiny bit uncomfortable. And it takes less than half a minute. While you're "legs up" on my exam table and I'm examining the top of your vagina, I'll take a sample of cells from your cervix by brushing across it with a little instrument specially made for this procedure.

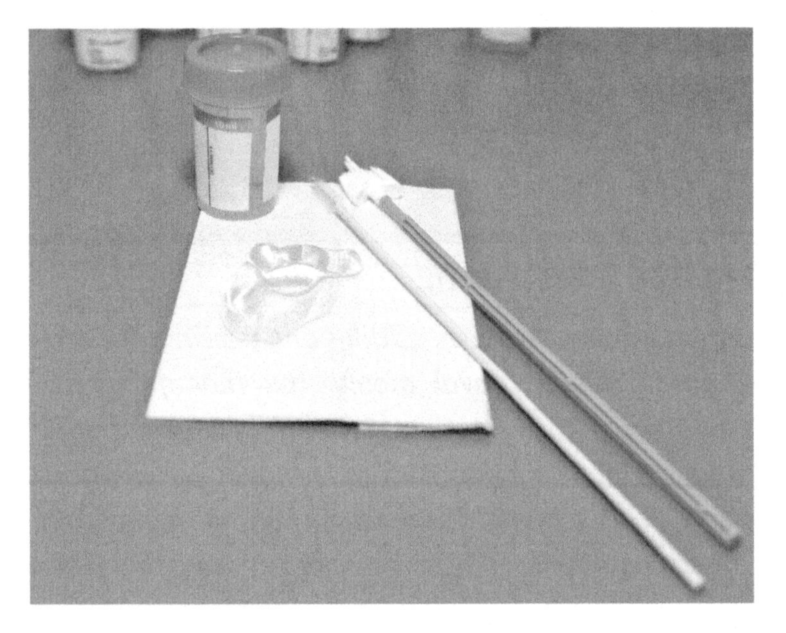

I'll place the smear of cervical cells into a vial of liquid preservative, which will be sealed and sent off to a pathology laboratory. At the laboratory, a technician will look at the cells under a microscope, note what is seen, and send back a report of the results. It may take several weeks before I receive the test results.

It's for Screening

Remember, your Pap test is a screening test. Here's the question it answers: does your cervix have normal cells or are the cells not normal? Pap test results try to categorize how worried we should be about your cervix. Mostly, they just alert your doctor to investigate further.

Your Pap test is a screening test for normal or abnormal cells.

Pap Test Results

Your Pap test results will come back from the laboratory with a report that reads either "normal" or "abnormal."

Cancer Scare Dilemma: "My Pap test came back 'normal.' Is this good news?"

If your lab report indicates normal results, it means no cell changes were found on your cervix. This result is good news; but you will still need to get your Pap tests in the future because, over time, new cell changes can form on your cervix.

Cancer Scare Dilemma: "My Pap test came back 'abnormal.' Do I have cancer?"

If your Pap test report from the pathology lab indicates abnormal cells, I will determine the best step to take next. An abnormal test result does not necessarily mean that cancer cells were found; there's no need to panic just because your report indicates abnormal changes. For sure though, an abnormal test result indicates that further testing or follow-up should be done.

ASC-US

One common abnormal Pap finding reads: Atypical Squamous Cells of Undetermined Significance (abbreviated ***ASC-US***). This finding simply means the cells look "funny," but we don't yet know whether we need to be worried about them; your cervical cells just look like they could be abnormal.

Coming to Terms

ASC-US is the abbreviation for a common abnormal Pap finding: Atypical Squamous Cells of Undetermined Significance.

An ASC-US finding does not make it clear whether the result is related to HPV. It could be related to life changes like pregnancy, menopause, or an infection.

I have heard other medical personnel comment, "It's just ASC-US," meaning they don't think it indicates a risk. However, it could indeed be serious (like carcinoma *in situ*, one step away from cancer) or not serious. We must do further investigation before making any judgments.

With ASC-US results, I commonly recommend looking for other types of vaginal infections (yeast, bacterial); looking at Ph imbalances; and looking for atrophic changes that can make your vagina and cervix dry, thin, and pale.

For most of my patients who receive abnormal Pap test results, I recommend a diagnostic test called a colposcopy.

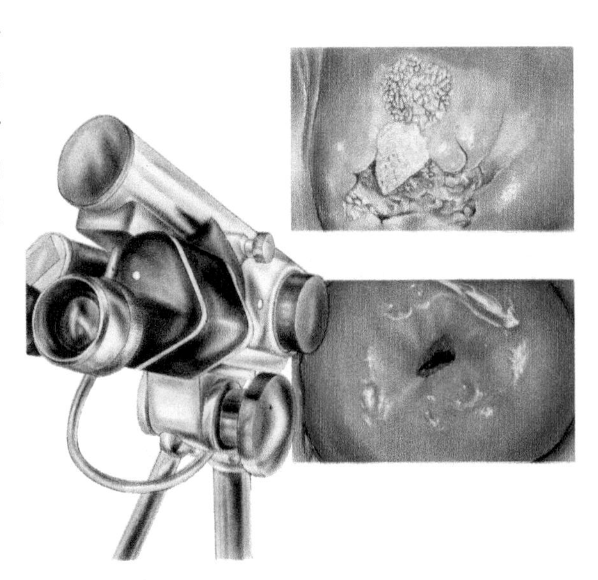

Cancer Scare Dilemma: "Colposcopy? That sounds ominous."

It's a tongue twister all right. But having a colposcopy doesn't mean something bad is about to happen. This in-office procedure is done to more closely examine your cervical tissue.

> **Coming to Terms**
>
> ***Colposcope***—Instrument named from root words colpos (vagina) and scope (view).

Remember, high-risk HPV and the cellular changes it causes are invisible to the naked eye until someone has advanced cancer. During your colposcopy, I employ techniques to make cellular changes visible.

We start this procedure with you in your "legs up" position. I'll place a speculum so that your cervix is visible. Then I'll swab a vinegar solution onto your cervix. This solution is a mild acid that turns any abnormal cells white so that I can see them. I'll look at your cervix under magnification with an instrument called a colposcope.

Once the white cells are visualized, I will take a small "pinch" biopsy of the most abnormal-looking area. Another sample will be taken from inside the canal of your cervix. This procedure often causes a sensation like menstrual cramps. I may put a topical agent on your cervix to stop any bleeding present after the biopsies. The specimens will be sent to a pathology laboratory to determine how severe the changes are on your cervix.

Cancer Scare Dilemma: "Will I be treated right away?"

After the pathology laboratory sends back your colposcopy results, I will take many factors into consideration as to what the next step should be. These factors include:

- Where were your abnormal cells found?
- How severe is the change?
- How long were abnormal cells present?
- What is your age?

Depending on your specific situation, we may or may not immediately treat precancerous cells. I will consult data sheets that analyze many factors which help determine when and how to treat precancer or unusual development or growth in the cervical area.

For patients younger than age twenty-five with mild changes, the recommendation might be to simply repeat their Pap tests on a schedule that will suit their individual situation.

Techniques for Treatment

When tests indicate treatment of a precancerous lesion, it is important to understand that no treatment can eradicate the cancer-causing virus (the unwelcome visitor, High-Risk Human Papilloma Virus) that caused normal cells on your cervix to turn abnormal. Once you contract HRHPV, you will always have that virus.

No treatment can eradicate the High-Risk Human Papilloma Virus.

Destroying Precancerous Cells

Some treatment therapies are intended to destroy precancerous cells, interrupting the progression toward cancer at that time. Cryotherapy (freezing) is one of several treatment techniques commonly used to destroy precancerous lesions. Others include chemotherapy, liquid acid solutions, or cautery to destroy tissue by burning. As the area heals, your tissue often grows back with normal architecture.

Surgical Treatment

Precancerous cells may be ***excised*** (surgically removed) by cutting them away. Common terms you might hear are: laser cone, cold knife conization, and LEEP. We'll focus on the most common surgical treatment (with the funny-sounding name), LEEP.

LEEP

A surgical therapy I perform in my office for removal of abnormal cells on the cervix is ***LEEP*** (short for loop electrosurgical excision procedure). This procedure removes abnormal tissue by cutting it away using a thin wire loop that carries an electrical current. During LEEP,

- the cervix is visualized using a speculum placed in the vagina,
- the area is numbed with a local anesthetic,
- the top skin layer of the cervix affected by precancer is shaved off using a hot wire, and
- the edges are cauterized to stop bleeding and to treat any abnormal cells that may not yet be visible.

About ninety percent of the time, LEEP will effectively remove precancerous cells, returning your Pap test to normal. If not, I may recommend another treatment.

Cancer Scare Dilemma:
"Will I get precancer again?"

I have heard patients say they were told that, once their precancer was treated, they would not get it back. That information is not true. The cancer-causing virus either continues to grow or goes dormant. If it starts to grow again later, you could have to start the process all over again.

You will need follow-up cervical cancer screening exams to detect when and if the virus starts growing again and if new precancerous changes occur.

This issue brings me to my last point:

Cervical Cancer Screening Guidelines

Did you know that, as of March 2012, the United States Preventive Services Task Force (USPSTF) and the American Cancer Society (ACS) no longer recommend having a Pap test annually?

Warning

The New NIH Screening Interval Guidelines May not Apply to You.

According to the National Cancer Institute at the National Institutes of Health (and I quote):

- *Cervical cancer screening, which includes the Pap test and HPV testing, is an essential part of a woman's routine health care because it can detect cancer or abnormalities that may lead to cancer of the cervix.*

- *Current guidelines recommend that women should have a Pap test every three years beginning at age twenty-one. These guidelines further recommend that women ages thirty to sixty-five should have HPV and Pap cotesting every five years or a Pap test alone every three years. Women with certain risk factors may need to have more frequent screening or to continue screening beyond age sixty-five.*
- *Women who have received the HPV vaccine still need regular cervical screening.*

Most women are not in the category for NIH screening interval guidelines.

You should note that, as a practical matter, the NIH screening interval guidelines are only appropriate for women at low risk with no history of high-risk HPV or abnormal Pap smears.

Although there may be some women whose history and current situations make them candidates for the new NIH guidelines, most women are not in that category. For example, if you have a new sexual partner, don't wait three to five years to get retested.

Based on Statistics

The new NIH screening interval guidelines are based on statistics.

I deal with women's lives daily, not statistics. As I noted before, I have seen women with no sign of precancerous changes on their cervix one year and carcinoma *in situ* the very next year.

Testing depends on each individual's particular risk situation.

Here is my personal observation: Is the NIH going to be the one to come inform my patients they have cervical cancer, which could have been prevented if they hadn't followed testing guidelines formulated on statistical data? Will statistical data matter to a woman when she is the one diagnosed with a preventable cancer, yet doctors didn't detect it in time?

Cancer Scare Dilemma: "How often should I get my Pap tests?"

The short answer is: as often as necessary to be sure you will be diagnosed with any changes in time for treatment of preventable cancer. It all depends on your particular risk situation.

The bottom line: You should discuss your situation with your gynecologist to determine the Pap screening interval that is right for you.

Newest Development—DNA Test for HRHPV

In April of 2014 the FDA approved a new DNA screening device for cervical cancer, the COBAS-HPV test. A cervical sample is collected in a similar fashion as liquid-based Pap tests, but the sample is screened for the presence of HRHPV types instead of looking for abnormal cells. As of the date of this book's publication, this test does not replace the Pap smear as the standard of care for cervical cancer screening. The full integration of new technology in healthcare always takes time. Watch for further developments.

Don't Stop Those Pap Tests Too Soon

New findings confirm that the age in life when cervical cancer peaks (the age at which women have the highest rate of cancer of the cervix) occurs at age sixty-five to sixty-nine.

Highest rates of cervical cancer occur at age 65 to 69.

So why do the NIH and others recommend stopping routine Pap tests on women at age sixty-five—right at the moment of their greatest need? The answer is: statistics. Those original studies based their recommendation on statistics that included women who have had hysterectomies. The new studies correct this statistical mistake, calculating the incidence of cervical cancer in the United States by including only women who actually have a cervix. Based on the latest evidence, I recommend that you continue your routine Pap screening past age 65.

On to the Hidden Truth

If you were a man and something had gone horribly wrong with the shaft of your penis, you wouldn't need someone to tell you about it, because your problem would be right there in plain sight.

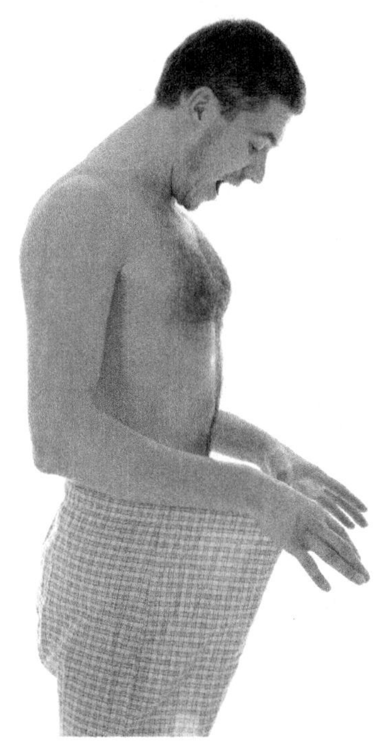

Not so with women's vaginal problems. Mother Nature tucked your vagina up inside you. Therefore, your Granny Vagina Dilemma might well have been a "hidden truth" that no one ever told you about. Women patients have voiced this complaint—Why didn't anyone ever tell me?—so many times that I felt compelled to include the whole next chapter, dedicated to answering your question.

Chapter Thirteen

Why Didn't Anyone Ever Tell Me?

Granny Vagina Dilemma:
"I've gone every year for my annual exam. Nobody ever told me I was getting a Granny Vagina."

"Was it a government conspiracy, something they don't want me to know?"

No, I doubt whether it was a government conspiracy. Do we really think the government knows about your Granny Vagina? Would they care if they did know?

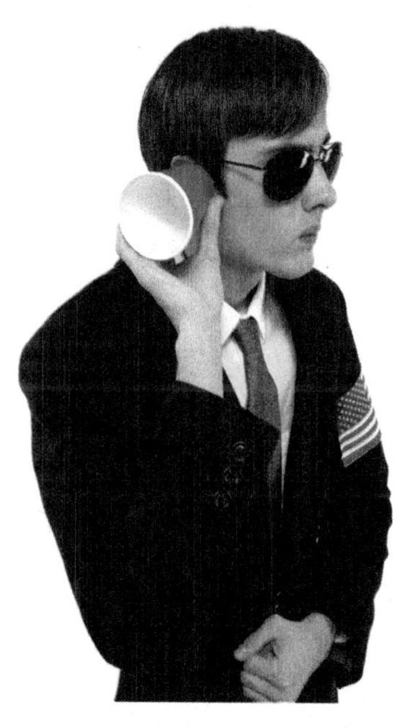

"Is Big Pharma deliberately trying to hide something from me?"

How about Big Pharma—now there's a real villain. The answer is: probably not. Nowhere in the pages of this book did we find evidence that the pharmaceutical industry has anything to gain from not telling you about your Granny Vagina. Pharmaceutical companies profit when you choose to buy their products; why should they try to hide your Dilemmas from you?

No Pharmaceutical $$$

No dollars from pharmaceutical companies were taken in making this book. The inclusion of product trademarks in this book does not imply endorsement.

"Do doctors know that I have Granny Vagina, but they won't tell me?"

Do doctors know but won't tell? Well, that situation is rarely, if ever, the case with doctors. But sometimes it does happen in real life with other people. Here's an example of someone who didn't tell what she knew:

Life Lesson: Don't Tell Everything You Know
My Granma was a sweet little lady. Everyone loved her. She was always looking for ways to stretch the food budget. Granma raised a big garden and the pressure cooker hissed away on the back burner of the kitchen stove as she toiled all summer to fill the shelves in the basement with rows and rows of canned fruit and vegetables.

One year a lady offered Granma all the windfalls on the ground underneath her apricot tree. Pailful

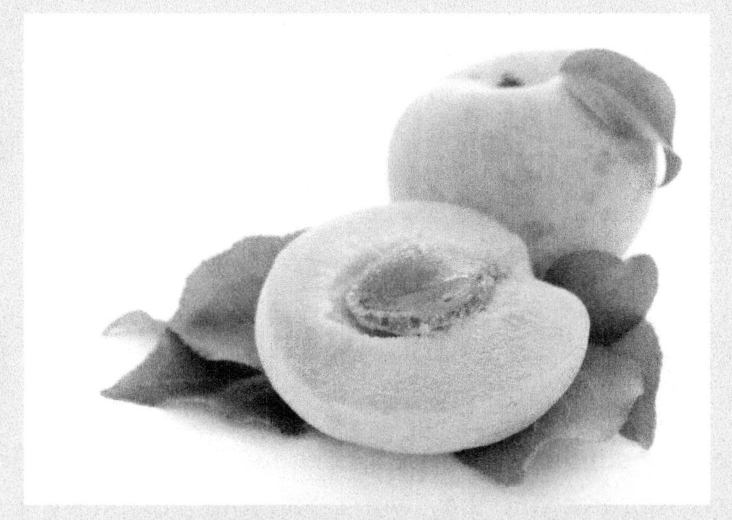

by pailful, Granma hauled those apricots home, canning up many jars of plump, beautiful yellow fruit. Soon she became famous for her apricot pies, always a big hit at church suppers. At home, Granma lined up all her grandkids and, with a big smile on her face, dished out slices of apricot pie all around.

Time takes its toll, and my beloved Granma eventually died. While Granma lay there in her coffin, with still the slightest little smile on her face, relatives reminisced about happy days gone by; someone mentioned those wonderful apricot pies.

"Oh," said Cousin Abby. "Do you mean those wormy apricots?" Abby had helped Granma can the apricots and she was the only one who knew Granma's secret.

It seems the reason so many apricots had fallen from the tree was because each one had a little worm inside. The worms were too difficult to pick out. Well, Granma wasn't going to let all those juicy apricots go to waste, and she figured a few well-cooked worms weren't going to hurt anybody. So, she just canned them up, worms and all. She added a drop of yellow food coloring to each jar, and those little worms turned yellow and blended right in with the fruit.

No wonder Granma served up her wormy apricot pies with a mischievous smile on her face. No one was the wiser. She knew but she didn't tell.

Now, do we suppose that doctors know all about your Granny Vagina symptoms but they won't tell you? Personally, I don't think that's the case. I'm passionate about what I do, and the medical profession abounds with doctors who also love their field of expertise. We're here to promote good health.

There are healthcare providers (usually gynecological surgeons) who have had extensive training in this area, and they take the time to do excellent pelvic examinations. How fortunate for you and your vagina if you have access to such a knowledgeable person!

"So, what's the answer? Why didn't anyone ever tell me?"

You may be shaking your head and saying, "I take good care of my health. I always get my regular check-ups. No one ever told me I was getting a Granny Vagina. Why didn't anyone ever tell me?" Simply stated, the answer may lie with whether the person doing your exam was genuinely knowledgeable about vaginas.

The person doing your exam should be genuinely knowledgeable about vaginas.

What Were They Looking For?

If you are developing Granny Vagina symptoms, and yet no one ever told you about the risks you face, it could be that you've been getting your exams from a healthcare provider who was focusing on something else, and not your possible vaginal problems.

Let's take a look at some of the people who do annual exams.

Your Family Doctor

Maybe you've been going to your general physician (also known as your family doctor) for your routine annual check-up. And you always thought this check-up included a good gynecological exam.

Did it?

Think back—did your doctor have to fit you into an already overbooked schedule? When your turn finally came, your private parts were probably looked at briefly, along with many other things. But no, a brief "Look-See" is not the same as a good gynecological exam.

A brief "Look-See" is not enough.

Your pelvic area is just one of many important body parts your family doctor will be considering in a routine exam. Starting somewhere in the vicinity of your eyes, the doctor will continue on down your body, checking you out.

But all too often, when your general physician reaches your pelvic area, "Legs up in these stirrups now," he or she may treat it like just another of the many areas to be given a brief visual screening: nothing more than inserting a speculum for a quick peek at your cervix. And while in there, a Pap smear to be sent off for a lab test.

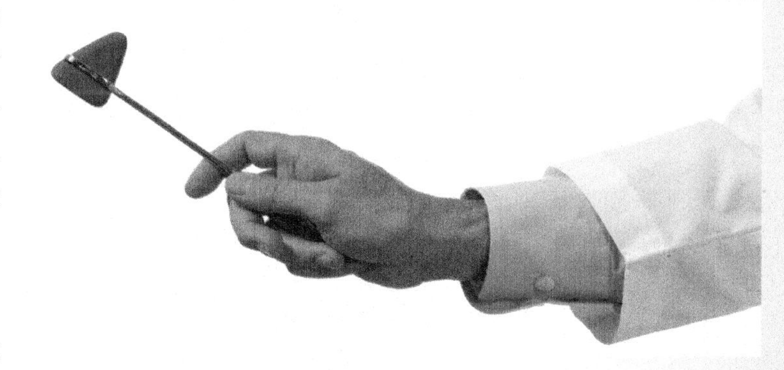

Then it's, "Legs down now. Sit up." A bonk

on the knees with a rubber hammer, a little more prodding and poking, and you're done.

Any questions? Your doctor might have been too busy to take the time to do a thorough vaginal exam unless you complained about something. If you don't offer any questions or concerns about your vagina, you're ready to put on your panties and go home.

All this happened without ever finding your Granny Vagina symptoms.

OB/GYN

Is your OB/GYN more OB than GYN?

The correct term for this medical specialty is Obstetrics and Gynecology. Medical school training and a residency in OB/GYN includes both:

- ***Obstetrics (OB)***—all about giving care to pregnant women and delivering their babies
- ***Gynecology (GYN)***—involving women's reproductive health

Each of these areas is vitally important in its own right. There are some colleges that consider splitting the specialty, making Obstetrics into one branch of medicine and Gynecology into a separate branch. Separating the two fields would allow in-depth training specific to the differing needs of women as they progress from their reproductive years into later life.

Traditionally, many doctors who practice Obstetrics and Gynecology will see patients in each category. That is, you can go to your local OB/GYN office for your prenatal care; then, when it's time, have the doctor deliver your baby; and later come back to the same doctor for your annual exams. But, is this schedule still the best idea?

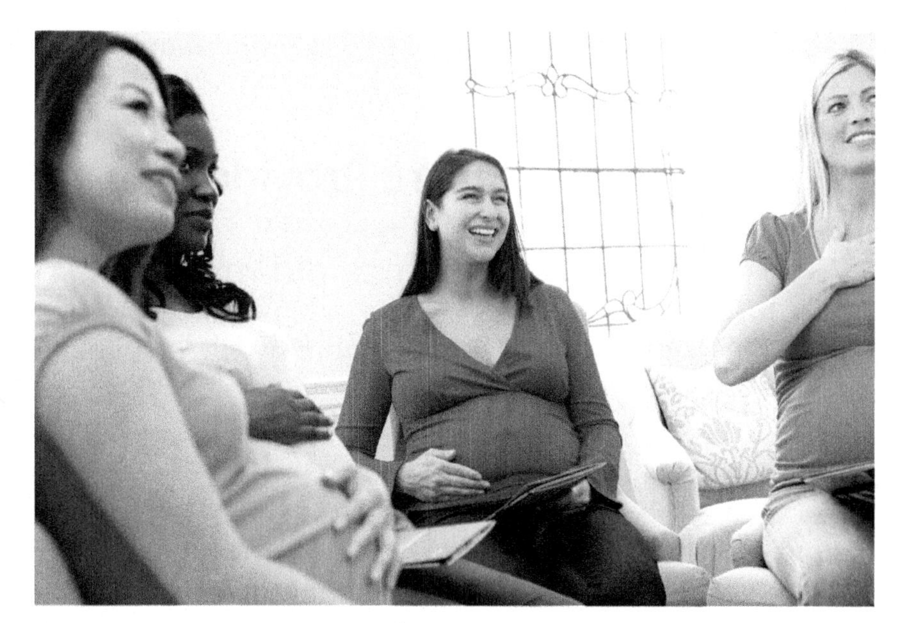

Take a look around your OB/GYN's waiting room:

- Does everyone else seem to be sprouting a Baby Bump?
- Was your appointment cancelled or postponed because your doctor was called to the hospital to deliver a baby?

Obstetrics is one of the most rewarding specialties in medicine; but it is also one of the busiest and most difficult. OB is an extremely time-consuming specialty, in itself. Doctors who devote most of their time to caring for pregnancies and delivering babies simply may not have the time (or the special training) to focus on your uterus when there isn't a baby growing in there.

Think back to your last annual exam with your OB/GYN. How much time was scheduled—fifteen minutes or less?

- If your doctor's schedule didn't allow enough time for a thorough pelvic exam;
- If your doctor knows all about "birthing babies" but has had no special training in Granny Vagina issues; then
- Your doctor might not have even paid attention to your Granny Vagina symptoms.

If that's the case, it's no wonder your OB/GYN never told you about your Granny Vagina.

Other Healthcare Providers

"Someone else in the office did my exam."

Your annual exam might have been carried out by someone who works under the supervision of your doctor. That's not necessarily a bad thing. The issue is: Was that person genuinely knowledgeable about vaginas?

Let's put it this way—can you expect a doctor who has had no special training in this area to have a staff of helpers who are any better prepared? If they're not, you had better look elsewhere.

A busy gynecologist with a well-run office will probably employ a whole staff of helpers. In addition to the office staff up front, the office could include midlevel providers such as:

- Medical assistants
- Physician assistants
- Nurse practitioners

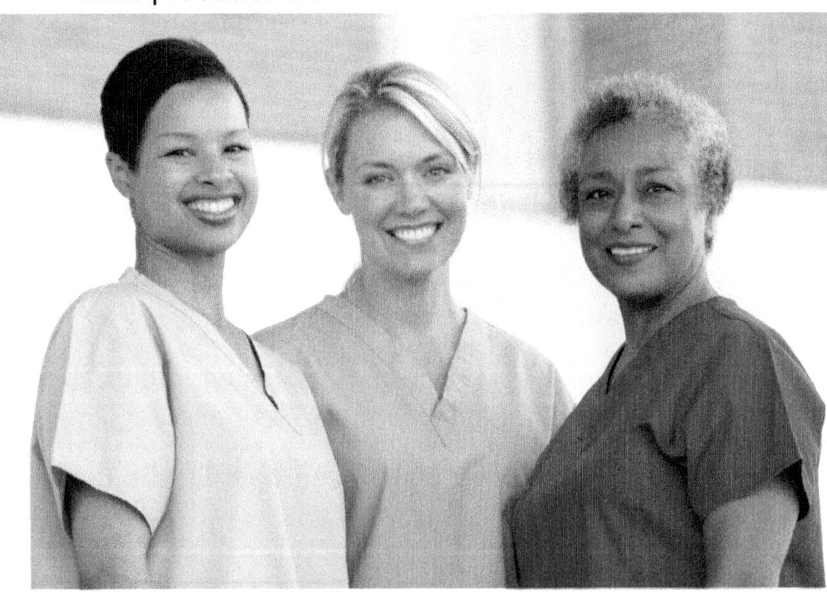

A well-trained professional midlevel provider can do an excellent job assisting your doctor. Your gynecologist may assign one of these professionals to carry out the screening portion of your annual exam.

There's a Right Way to Do It

A good gynecologist will prepare her entire team to be specialists in this area. Knowledgeable midlevel providers can perform the screening portion of your exam and then pass this information on to your gynecologist.

Looking for Signs

There's not a little flashing arrow down there warning "CAUTION!" "Granny Vagina in Progress!" It takes the right person with the right training to know which symptoms to look for, what to ask, and how to decipher any signs that warn of impending Granny Vagina trouble.

There's no CAUTION sign down there.

Quality Time

In my office, after you are finished with the routine screening portion of your exam, it's time for you and me to spend some quality time together. I'm the one who will be the bearer of good news if your vagina is pink and perky, or bad news if you show signs of a Granny Vagina.

Maybe you haven't yet noticed any symptoms, but if indications of Granny Vagina are there, I'll tell you. Then we can make another appointment for you to come in for further diagnoses.

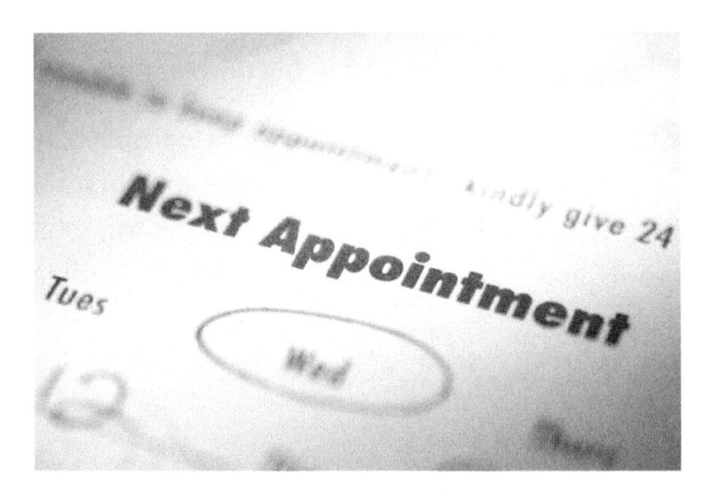

Diagnosis Is Key

Proper diagnosis is key to treating pelvic support problems. The exact cause of the problem must be found before the best treatment can be given. Being open about your symptoms can help me find the exact cause.

Because vaginal problems are my specialty, I focus on Granny Vaginas with every patient who comes to see me.

Coming Up: Step-by-Step

In the next chapter we'll go through a step-by step description of what happens during a good annual wellness/pelvic screening examination.

Chapter Fourteen

Your Annual Wellness/Pelvic Screening Examination

First of All—What to Call It

You may simply think of it as your "annual," that time each year when you pay a visit to your gynecologist to have your lady-parts checked, make sure you are in generally good health, and see to it that your tests and prescriptions are up-to-date.

This exam is known by a whole bunch of names—annual pelvic examination, annual pelvic screening examination, yearly medical examination, annual check-up, routine healthcare visit. Medicare introduced the term "Annual Wellness Visit." Many insurance companies have their own designation.

An Exam by Any Other Name ...

No matter what it's called, an annual exam is a good thing. Patients who follow a personal wellness plan, including a thorough check-up every year, will reduce the odds of developing expensive and debilitating conditions over their lifespan.

Let's Call it Something

In my office, I've coined the term *Annual Wellness/Pelvic Screening Examination.* That elaborate title seems to cover all the bases. Throughout this book, I've shortened it to your "annual exam."

I'll call it your "annual exam."

How Long Will It Take?

With some doctors, your examination might take as little as ten to twenty minutes. In my office, I schedule a half hour to forty-five minutes for a full annual exam. For patients with known health problems, I will take more time. You'll need less time if you are not due for a full exam; for example, if all you need is a routine follow-up Pap test or a routine post-operative check.

Your Insurance Company Defines What's Done

Maybe you're thinking, "I'll go in for my annual exam, and while I'm there, I'll have Dr. King take care of this other problem." You're hoping that, after I examine you, I will also (for example) take an ultrasound or discuss your need for hormones. I wish it were possible, but unfortunately it's not!

With many insurance providers, only the screening portion of your annual exam is covered without cost to you, and insurance covers the screening portion only if no other procedures are done in the same visit. If screening indicates that you need other procedures, we will make another appointment for you to come back.

No other procedures should be done in the same visit.

Follow Those Codes

For insurance purposes, there are universal codes assigned to all the known medical conditions. There are also codes assigned to each and every medical procedure. There are thousands of these codes. The code assigned to an annual exam is different from codes assigned to other medical conditions and symptoms. As physicians, we are bound by law to assign codes truthfully and accurately for our diagnoses and for procedures we perform.

For your exam, I will submit one code to your insurance company, indicating that I performed only one procedure (screening) on that visit.

Not Included in Your Annual Exam

Treatment for:

- *Bleeding problems, irregular menstrual periods*
- *Pain*
- *Cysts*
- *Infections*

Consultation for:

- *Hormone evaluation*
- *Libido issues*

Screening and Another Procedure Together?

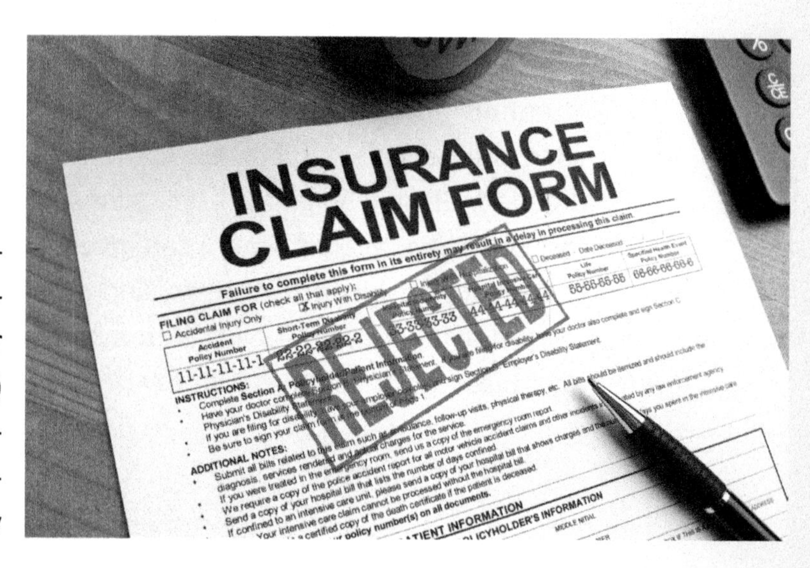

If your doctor performs another procedure for you (for instance, ultrasound) along with your annual exam, your insurance company might pay for neither. Maybe in years past this situation was not the rule, but with many insurance companies, that's the way it is now. Why? Talk to your insurance company. They make the rules about what they will pay and when.

If your insurance company denies coverage, you will end up paying for your exam (which would otherwise have been covered) and the additional procedure, as well. In my office, we found out about this denial the hard way.

Case in Point

I remember the time I was doing an annual exam on one of my patients when I noticed a large, dark, dangerous-looking mole on her back. I was afraid it might be skin cancer and thought it was imperative to take that mole off immediately; I wouldn't let her leave until I did so. Because the lesion removal was done in the same visit with her exam, however, her insurance company refused to cover anything, and the patient had to pay out-of-pocket for her exam and for having her mole removed.

You May Have to Come Back

If your annual exam indicates a problem that needs further attention (for example, your menstrual periods are too heavy, your uterus is enlarged, or—heaven forbid—evidence of the dreaded Granny Vagina), I will schedule another appointment for you. Then, at that time, I can investigate your problem more specifically, order further tests, and get you started on the road toward living longer, feeling better, and looking lovely with the healthiest, prettiest vagina in town.

A Brief Description of the Basics

I find that women are often confused about what their annual exam routinely covers and what it does not. So, here is an overview of the basic things you can expect when you come in once a year for your annual exam.

What's Included in Your Annual Exam?

Well, There's Screening

Your annual exam is a screening evaluation. Its purpose is to simply look for any signs or symptoms of impending problems in a patient who otherwise shows no symptoms.

An annual exam starts by assuming you're healthy. I will start at the top of you and work my way down, screening out problems that are not showing up (no sign of this problem, no symptom of that disorder), all the while looking closely for anything that's not as it should be.

If You're a New Patient

If you're new to my office, I will need background and insurance information (and incidentally, if you've not been seen by my practice for more than three years, you are again considered to be a new patient here).

It is also important to record information about your menstrual periods:

- How old were you when they started?
- How far apart?
- How long do they last?

- Are they heavy or light?
- Any cramping?
- Are you in need of any birth control?

Medical Assistant Gets You Ready

My medical assistant will take all your vital signs and note them in your record. She will also review your medical history with you and update your chart with anything current that needs to be added.

Urine Sample

You will be asked to leave a urine sample. Simply pee in a cup; we put a dipstick into your urine sample. The stick has squares with different reagents. These reagents change color when they come in contact with chemicals in the urine. I will review the results with you later in your examination.

My medical assistant will give you a gown and instruct you to undress; then you will be ready to sit up on the exam table, with a white sheet modestly covering your nether region.

I Begin the Exam

Your Vital Signs are Important

I need to review all your vital signs, typically:

- Height—are you losing height?
- Weight—is it changing, are you over, under, or maintaining proper weight?
- Blood pressure—too high, too low?
- Pulse—too fast?

If your vital signs are out of order, this situation indicates something amiss, and I will look for the reason.

Medical History

Then I will review your medical history: anything new since your last visit—allergies, surgeries, medical conditions, medications, social history (marriage, smoking, drugs), and family history. What am I looking for? Changes: for example, a new medical issue with a close family member. If a relative close to you has developed cancer, we may need to see you more often and modify your screening schedule.

I'm looking for changes in your medical history.

I will review your age-appropriate screenings (Pap test, bone density, mammogram, and colonoscopy), and I'll look to see if you are current with your vaccinations (for teenagers, Gardasil; for patients over sixty, shingles and flu vaccine).

Finally, I will ask if you have any concerns about health issues we should give specific attention to.

Urinalysis

I will review the results of your urine test. If no problems are indicated, the urine sample will be thrown away. If, however, I see evidence of diabetes or kidney disease, I will order further screening.

If the results of the dipstick test indicate a urinary tract or bladder infection, I will ask, "Are you experiencing any symptoms of a bladder infection, like frequency or urgency?" I will send a sample to be cultured to determine the exact cause.

The specific gravity of your urine sample will show evidence of any dehydration. By observing the concentration of your urine, I will be able to see whether you are dehydrated.

On to the Physical Part of Your Exam

I will examine you starting at the top; then I'll work my way down. I will be noting your general appearance: are your eyes white? do you appear happy or sad? do you appear tired?

Thyroid, Lymph Nodes

I will gently feel your ***thyroid*** (a butterfly-shaped gland that sits between and just above your collar bones, behind your long neck muscles). I will ask you to swallow, which pulls the thyroid gland up through my fingers, so that I will be able to feel any enlargement or nodules. I will also feel for swollen lymph nodes in the neck and above the collar bones.

> **Coming to Terms**
>
> Your ***thyroid*** is a butterfly-shaped gland that sits between and just above your collar bones, behind your long neck muscles.

Thyroid problems are common and may cause weight gain, or irregular or heavy menstrual periods. If I find nodules, I will run thyroid studies and refer you for an ultrasound examination. A more extensive head and neck evaluation will be done if you are having other complaints.

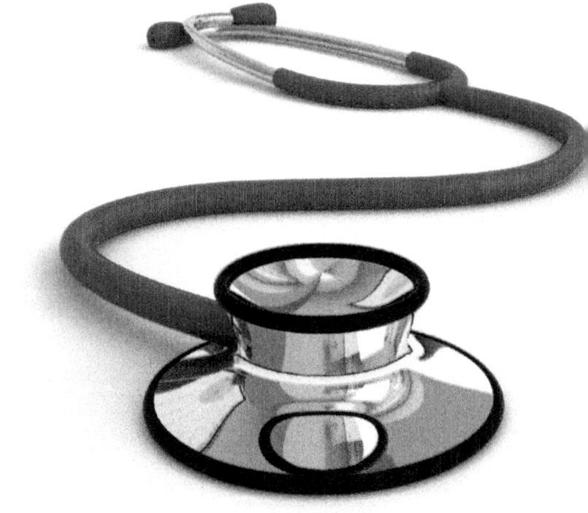

Heart, Lungs

I will use the stethoscope to listen to your lungs, where I'll check for wheezing or other abnormal breathing sounds. I'll also listen to your heart to check your heart rate, to determine if the beats are regular in timing, and to tell if you have a heart murmur.

I am amazed by the number of times I have been the first doctor to mention a patient's heart murmur or to recommend that it be investigated. Too often, patients were told their murmur is ***benign*** (not dangerous), without proper evaluation. One of my patients had a loud heart murmur but had been told there was no problem, when she actually needed a heart valve replacement. I never conclude something is benign without at least doing further testing.

Breast Exam

I will do a thorough breast exam, using gentle pressure of my fingers to feel for lumps in the breast tissue, including the part extending into the area of your armpit. I will also teach you how to do a proper self-exam, which you should do monthly at home. This examination is important because most breast lumps are actually found by women, themselves.

You should do self-exams monthly.

Abdomen

Routine examination of the abdomen includes feeling for masses that would indicate liver enlargement or hernias, as well as listening to the abdomen for abnormal intestinal sounds.

Gynecological Part of Your Exam

As a gynecologist, I will give special attention to examination of your pelvic area.

Visual Inspection

Legs up now, it's time for my visual inspection of your vulva and external labia. I will be looking for any lumps, bumps, growths, rashes, or discharge. Also:

- Do your labia look healthy or are they elongated, discolored, or saggy?
- Does the opening to your vagina gape open? Can I see right into your vagina without first separating your labia minor?
- How about the area between the opening of the vagina and the opening of the anus? Is it short or does it have scars from childbirth?
- Are there any obvious hemorrhoids?

The Speculum Exam

The speculum is a two-sided metal instrument that I will gently insert into your vagina to open it and hold it open while I inspect your intra-vaginal structures.

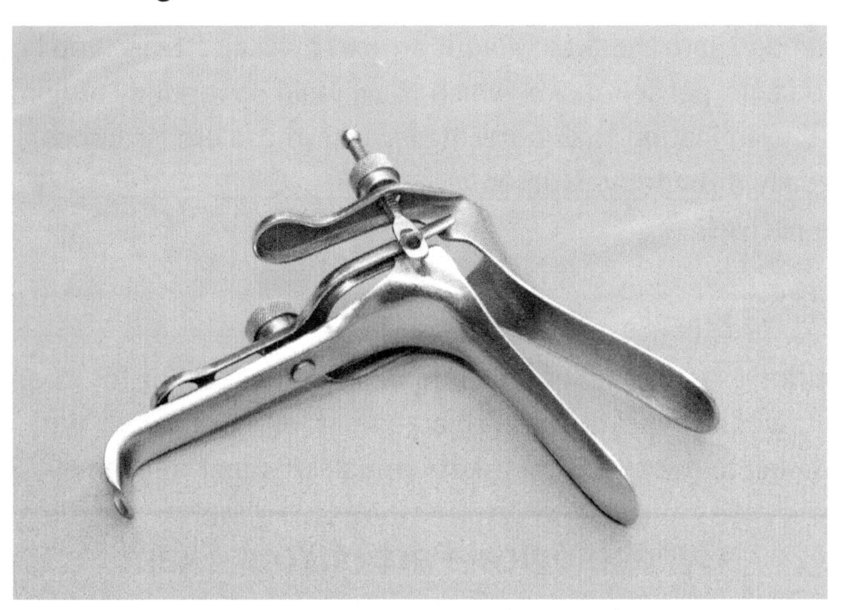

At this point, I may undertake cervical cancer screening tests, according to the screening schedule that is appropriate for you. I will consider your risk factors that we discussed in "You've Gone Viral."

A swab of the vaginal discharge may be obtained. I will evaluate the color, consistency, and amount of discharge. This sample will be used to check for sexually transmitted diseases (***gonorrhea*** and ***chlamydia***). If necessary, I will do a culture, or look at the discharge under a microscope.

> **Coming to Terms**
>
> ***Gonorrhea*** and ***chlamydia*** are sexually transmitted diseases.

Next, while gently pulling the speculum back out, I will inspect your vaginal tissue. I'll be looking at the quality of the ***vaginal mucosa*** (tissue), and checking to see if the color is pink, if it is moist, and if it has rugations (folds). I'll be able to determine whether there is prolapsed tissue.

For women who have had children, I will check to see if the vagina is stretched and baggy.

Exam for Pelvic Organ Prolapse

The regular, two-sided speculum is actually a hindrance when examining you for pelvic organ prolapse, because it covers up and distorts the anatomy of your vagina.

A regular speculum is a hindrance when examining for pelvic organ prolapse.

Instead, I use a specially modified instrument that will allow me to get a clear view of each wall of the vagina individually. This way, I will be able to diagnose whether any organs are bulging into your vagina, how many organs are affected, and to what extent. During this part of the exam, I will often have you bear down to see if the vaginal walls protrude down farther.

To assist me in diagnosing bladder problems, I may ask you to strain or cough during your exam to see if you leak urine. Your bladder may look as if it is in its proper position until you bear down, whereupon it may move or significantly rotate down your vagina. I may perform an examination for rectal prolapse, as well.

Palpation

Palpation is a medical term for examination using gentle pressure of the fingers to check for abnormalities. I will place two fingers of one hand into your vagina and my other hand on your abdomen. By squeezing my fingers together, I will be able to feel your uterus and ovaries for size, shape, and discomfort. If I feel nodules behind your cervix, this finding could indicate ***endometriosis***, a condition in which the endometrial tissue is present in the ovaries or elsewhere in your body.

Coming to Terms

The medical term for examination using gentle pressure of the fingers to check for abnormalities is ***palpation***.

Endometriosis is a condition in which endometrial tissue, which normally lines only the uterus, is present in the ovaries or elsewhere in your body.

I might ask you to squeeze down and do a Kegel exercise while I palpate in order to assess your vaginal muscle tone. I will determine the size of your vaginal opening by stretching my two fingers apart. Prior to vaginal delivery of babies, the opening is usually snug to two fingers. After vaginal deliveries, stretching of three to five finger-widths is common.

We're Nearly Finished

Details Noted

A great deal of what I will be looking for and feeling comes automatically to me after having been in practice for nearly twenty years. Although I might not tell you every single thing I'm screening for as we go along ("Now I'm doing ... " "Now I'm looking for ... "), I will be paying attention to details in every area, noting any signs or symptoms of impending problems. I will be screening out problems that are not showing up, as well as closely looking for anything that's not as it should be.

Much of your annual exam will happen without your even being aware.

Let's Sit Down and Review

When I've completed all the areas of your screening, I'll ask you to get dressed and I will come back into the exam room to talk with you about what I've seen. It's time to sit down and review:

- Are there recommendations for additional screening tests, such as a mammogram, blood chemistry, health screening profile, or colonoscopy?
- Were there any unusual findings?
- What additional evaluations may be needed (ultrasound, diagnostic blood work)?
- Do you need a refill for any prescriptions?
- Are over-the-counter supplements recommended?

Your Questions and Concerns

Now is the time to make sure I have addressed all your questions and concerns. You should feel free to confide whatever is on your mind.

My goal is for you to be happy you came in, and for you to leave feeling reassured that you have had a thorough and productive annual wellness/ pelvic screening examination.

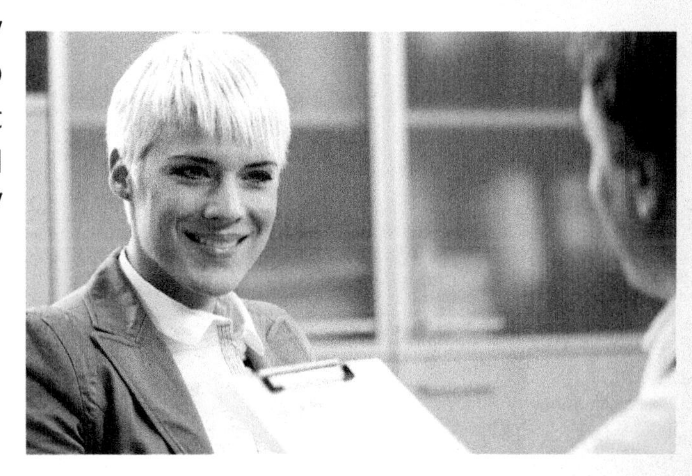

One Final Thought

Farewell, Readers, You've Inspired Me!

To all the women I've worked with in the course of my practice, "Thank you!" You've truly inspired me.

To all the women who read this book, I trust that you now have the power to become informed patients, to know what's normal, what's not normal, and to take greater control of changes to your vagina throughout your lifetime.

Together, we can make the world more beautiful—one vagina at a time.

Interview with the Author

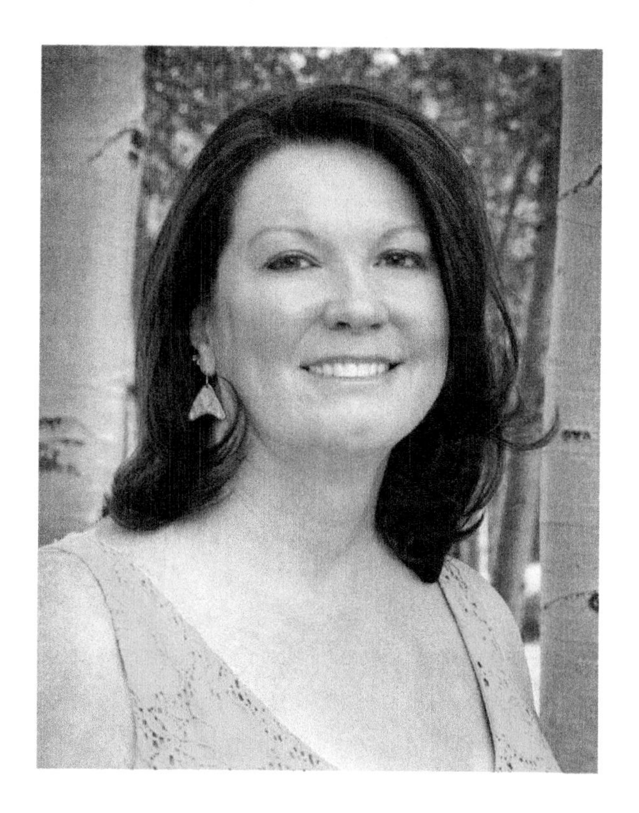

Who says a book has to be dull and boring, laden with medical jargon, in order to describe some of womanhood's most pressing problems? The author of *Legs Up!* has chosen a unique approach—speaking directly to readers in the same light-hearted conversational voice she uses with her patients every day.

By Ruth Ann Schneider

Dr. Gail King paid me the honor of sharing her manuscript before publication. I was struck by the complexity of the subject; I never would have guessed that vaginas could fill a whole book.

Dr. King is a woman of many talents. She built her career with a clear goal in sight, all the while taking on creative ideas and setting new precedents along the way.

From her office in Aspen, Colorado, the author generously found time to describe the inspiration she gets from her patients, and to share her personal journey, while offering some insights on leaving the well-worn path.

Let's start with your book. You begin with a terribly graphic picture of a woman's uterus hanging out of her vagina.
Well, that's real life, so why try to hide it? I took that picture myself. It is an unretouched picture of one of my patients with a prolapsed uterus. I want to let my readers know just how ghoulish things can get if they don't take care of their vaginas. Someone suggested that I put this picture on the cover of my book. But I think that if I did, bookstores might hide it away in their pornography section.

All women have vaginas. Why isn't there more information about this subject available to us?
It's not so much a matter of whether the information exists. It's out there, just generally unavailable, buried in textbooks and scattered among onerous medical articles. With a lot of digging around, women could find a little bit of information here and an explanation hidden away there—assuming they knew what to look for in the first place.

There's never been another single source of information on vaginas that goes into this level of detail. That's why I decided to change the situation. I said to myself why not write a practical book that brings vaginas out in the open (figuratively, of course).

Why did you decide to address such a serious theme as vaginal problems within such a light-hearted format?
I want my readers to relate to real-life issues that my patients are experiencing. Many women who will read this book have already encountered some of these problems with their own vaginas, or they probably know someone in their family, or perhaps friends, with similar experiences. That's why I decided to do something new—write about real-life issues in a real-life way.

But, of course, even though I've chosen an upbeat, fun format, these are actual health risks we're talking about. So my advice is always serious.

The story about the women in the kitchen discussing their stretched-out vaginas was very realistic. Were you inspired by anything similar that really happened?
No. Many women I know would never, ever let their guard down and be that open with each other, and that's too bad. I just dreamed up the idea of putting it into a fictional story, imagining what would happen if women dared to tell the truth about their stretched-out vaginas.

As for real-life women who are questioning whether they can ever bring themselves to be open about their sexual issues, it's easy to get caught up in fear. They're afraid to bring their sexual issues out in the open. My advice: Try discussing your feelings with your gynecologist, and there's a good chance you will be glad you did.

How do you relate to women who are having these Vagina Dilemmas?
Here is how I relate: I've had many of the Dilemmas that I write about in the book. I was already a graduate medical student in gynecology before a doctor asked me if sex was tight enough. I hadn't given it a second thought before then. I just accepted that my vagina was all stretched out because my body wasn't

the same after having children. I didn't know my vagina could be tightened.

I know from experience the issues childbearing can lead to. I had three babies vaginally; one was almost nine and a half pounds. My childbearing led to a rectocele, where my rectum bulged into my vagina. When the rectocele started causing symptoms, I had it fixed. But after my surgery, I was writhing in pain. At that point I thought surely this trauma doesn't have to be the way it is for us women. I was determined not to do that to my patients. Now I administer a pudendal nerve block that keeps surgery patients numb for eighteen to twenty-four hours, with adequate pain management afterwards.

Hormones are another example; I admit my bias towards them. They suddenly became important to me as I entered that stage of life. I'm not a man who will never know hot flashes. And I'm not young, fresh out of medical school, where there isn't time for an in-depth study of hormones. When I began experiencing hormonal fluctuations, I took an interest to go and learn about hormonal health and to get an education far beyond that provided for me in my medical school training.

Over the course of your career, what have you learned about patient concerns?

When a woman comes in to see me, I make it a point to listen to what is bothering her. In addition to what I may find medically urgent, I always want to be sure I adequately evaluate and address each patient's primary concern. If I don't address her primary concern, then I have failed her.

Once I get to know my patients and they trust me, I find they are honest with their feelings and their issues. Being a gynecologist, I'm privileged to have my patients feel comfortable enough to share intimate experiences and concerns with me.

Why use this book as a vehicle to tell about vaginal issues? Why not medical journal articles or other traditional publications?
This information is what my patients ask for. I wanted to write about real women with real problems, and I thought the best way to do it was to create a book written in the friendly language that I use with my patients. I intentionally did not write it as if it were a medical text, with page after page of dull facts, a boring volume of everything there is to know about procidentia and cystourethoceles. The story I was interested in telling was set in my office.

Granny Vagina problems have always been a taboo subject; women have just taken it for granted that bad things happen down there. As a result, many of my patients were taken by surprise when they learned about what's going on inside them and how we can go about fixing their problems. There's no reason why women shouldn't be comfortable talking about their vaginas. Let's get the discussion started!

What do you hope will be the "take-away" for your readers?
I hope they will enjoy reading this book. My intent is to connect emotionally. I hope it will create dialog so that women can openly talk about their vaginas and about sex—where one lady can bring up the subject and it will become the topic of conversation.

I also hope readers will gain a new way of communicating with healthcare workers. In the introduction, I recommend that every woman keep a copy of this book tucked in the drawer with her undies to refer to over time as vaginal issues arise. I also think it would be a great idea for readers to leave an extra copy at the front desk in their healthcare provider's office. The office staff will learn about their vaginas, and you can bet it will filter back to those persons who do annual exams.

Moving on to your career, when and why did you decide to become a physician? What other career path might you have followed?
As a five-year-old child, I used to "help" my father in his veterinary office. While he did surgery on cats and dogs, I stood on a stool and cut stitches. Way back then I decided: I want to be a doctor and do surgery, but I want to do it on people, not animals. I never seriously considered any other career. I found that my fascination with medicine never waned. It's my calling.

How would you describe your journey through your medical education? Was it clear sailing or were there some storm clouds along the way?
There were people along the way who were less than encouraging. For instance, I spent my sophomore year of high school in Germany as an exchange student. When I returned to my hometown high school, the guidance counselor was all confused because I had taken a non-traditional path. Because she didn't know how to translate my German school classes, she told me I could just drop out and take a job at McDonald's, rather than pursue a medical career.

Did that episode upset you? Did it make you want to quit your dream?
It might have upset me at the time, but it was irrelevant in the long run. I've always loved medicine so the thought never crossed my mind to detour into something else. I don't have time to dwell on those people in my life who don't understand my motivation. I've refused to let my own goals go by the wayside just because somebody else thought something different. And now I'm a board-certified gynecological surgeon.

Where did you attend medical school?
I applied for early admission at the University of Colorado School of Medicine at Denver. Early admission means that if they accept you early, you agree to attend there and not go somewhere else.

The school informs you by registered letter. One day I found a notice in my mailbox: the mailman had a registered letter I would have to sign for, but he didn't bring the letter to my door. I grabbed the notice and ran around my neighborhood to find that mailman because I couldn't wait until the next day to find out. (Yes, I was accepted.)

You were one of very few women who had children while they were in medical school.

My husband and I started our family while I was a pre-med student. I was six months pregnant with my second child when I interviewed for medical school. I remember I wore a teal maternity dress because I refused to wear the traditional black business suit. I didn't want to put my life on hold for medical school; I didn't want to be an old mother.

Having three children along the way proved to be an advantage for me. Medical students could study twenty-four hours a day, seven days a week and still fret that they needed to study more. By having a family, I was able to turn off when I came home. I became a mommy. It made me more effective in my studying because I had to be. Actually, research shows that college students who are involved in activities have to be more efficient, more focused on their studies. It makes them better students.

While I was a medical student, I also took on the additional responsibly of serving on the admissions committee because I knew I could bring a distinctive perspective to that process. I liked diversity—people who had real-life experience prior to applying. I gave consideration to people who had not taken the traditional path, those applicants who had interesting journeys. I, too, was taking the path less trodden.

How did you happen to come to Aspen?

After residency, my family and I moved to Noblesville, Indiana, where I practiced obstetrics and gynecology for nine years. It was a great place for the kids while they were young. Then the mountains called, and I relocated back to Colorado. I've never regretted it.

It's beautiful here in Aspen. Where else in the world would you want to live? Also, Aspen is progressive; the population is extremely health minded. When I was looking around at my options, I decided I liked Aspen and thought wouldn't it be wonderful if I could set up a successful practice here. No contacts, didn't know anyone. No foot in the door here to get me started. I could have taken a job that was more secure, joined an ongoing practice somewhere else. But—did this situation ever happen to you?—I said to myself, if I don't try it now, right now, I'll always wonder: What if I had tried? Could it have worked out? I was afraid that if I didn't at least try this venture, I would always regret it. So, I came to Aspen, and it's been even more fantastic than I ever dreamed it would be.

Looking at your practice, I see you've been going in some new directions.
People say, "Oh, I didn't know you did that." I do lots of new things. One of my personality traits is: I am a learner. I love learning new things. I think a doctor should continually learn. Keep up in your own area, and always have at least a working knowledge of most aspects of medicine, not just your specialty, so that you can help guide patients in the right direction.

When did you begin to be creative with new ideas, new things to use in your practice?
You know, while you're getting through medical school, there are very few independent decisions to make because the course is set out for you: what prerequisites you need to take, what exams to pass. It's regimented, and you experience the sensation of being herded like cattle through the process. I never stopped to contemplate writing a book, inventing a new procedure, leaving that well-worn path, until being in private practice.

Now I take a fresh look at everything I do. I'm constantly asking myself how I can improve, do something better so that it becomes more effective. That's how I came up with the idea for Vaginal Regenalift™.

Tell me more about Vaginal Regenalift™.
Vaginal Regenalift is my own trademarked procedure that uses platelet-rich-plasma (PRP). During surgery I collect about four ounces of my patient's own blood and process it in a special machine that separates red blood cells from the plasma, or serum, the red cells float in. Then I extract the layer that is rich in platelets. These components aggregate to form clotting. They also contain growth factors and signaling factors that signal the body to bring in the immune system to start the repair process. I reinject this platelet-rich-plasma into the repair site. It jump starts and enhances the healing process. It also decreases the risk of infection. I have noticed remarkable healing in my treated patients.

You say you use a laser in your surgeries. That technique sounds considerably "cutting edge" (pardon the pun).
You're right. I completed training with Dr. David Matlock, a gynecologist in California who is a recognized expert in the field of laser surgery. He pioneered a whole new method of using laser surgery to tighten and support the vagina. Dr. Matlock's patented process is called ***Laser Vaginal Rejuvenation,*** or ***LVR*** for short. I'm a certified associate of his Laser Vaginal Rejuvenation Institute of America.

I use a laser to do cutting and dissecting in my surgeries. It's a special laser, which is extremely gentle on tissue. There are many advantages. The laser is a precision cutting instrument. I can control it with pinpoint accuracy. Because it minimizes blood loss and swelling, laser surgery allows the body to heal rapidly. My patients can resume their daily activities in a short period of time.

Anything innovative coming up on the horizon for you?
I'm glad you asked me that question. Right now is such an exciting time to be involved on new frontiers in medicine; there are so many new doorways opening. To complement my gynecology practice, I recently completed my fellowship in a different area—antiaging and regenerative medicine. Antiaging medicine looks at how each patient's health trends over time. With that knowledge, problems can be headed off at the pass, before they become full blown.

Medical technology is moving away from just treating and managing symptoms (the disease model) to understanding the underlying root causes of illness and treating at that level. Many illnesses have toxins as their root cause. With our knowledge of the body's cellular and DNA components expanding so rapidly, we now understand therapeutic treatments that detox at the cellular and DNA level, while restoring the cells' proper phosphotidal balance. I liken it to an oil change in your car, except it's for every cell in your body.

I am co-founder of Regen Aspen, an advanced regenerative medical center, along with Dr. Fouad Ghaly, one of the most influential physicians working in the field of regenerative medicine. This specialty offers many state-of-the-art options: adult stem cell banking, telomere length testing, micronutrient and toxicity profiles, platelet-rich-plasma therapies, and EECP (enhanced extracorporeal counter pulsation), to name a few. Visit the website http://www.regenaspen.com for more information.

Finally, just for fun, where would you like to practice in your fantasy future?
I've heard there are some countries where vaginal rejuvenation is universal, where wives get their vaginas rebuilt after every child. Granny Vagina Dilemmas are routinely addressed. My fantasy would be to move there and do vaginal repairs all day long.

*Interviewer **Ruth Ann Schneider** is an attorney and author, currently retired and living in Florida.*

Appendix

Demystify Your Female Anatomy

Organs for Reproduction

Your lady-parts (organs for reproduction of our species) are nestled inside your pelvis.

Here are the various parts of your anatomy that connect together to make up your female sex apparatus.

Uterus

Your most important reproductive organ is your ***uterus***. It's that richly-lined cavity where a baby develops and is nourished during pregnancy.

Ovaries

At the top of your uterus, your ***fallopian tubes*** deliver ***ovum*** (tiny reproductive cells also called eggs) that are produced in female organs known as your ***ovaries***. The ovaries are found inside your abdomen and are attached to the uterus by a ligament.

Cervix

Cervix is the medical term for the lower, narrow end of the uterus. It is the part of your uterus sticking down into the vagina that dilates when you are in labor. It's also where we take a Pap test. (***Pap test*** is the common term for the Papanicolaou test, used to detect cervical cancer early.)

Vagina

From your cervix, your ***vagina*** (a hollow, muscular tube about three to seven inches long) forms a pathway to the outside of your body. The walls of your vagina are layered with muscle and connective tissue.

Vulva

The opening to your vagina is visible from outside; the folds of your ***vulva*** protect it. The outer folds of your vulva are ***labia***, often referred to as ***"lips."***

This picture shows how your uterus, cervix, vagina and vulva are connected together.

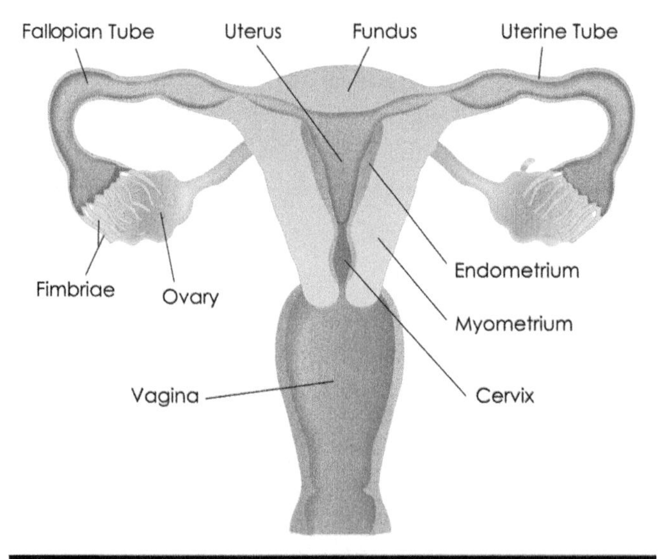

Share the Space

Sharing space in your pelvic cavity, near your reproductive organs, are other organs that have nothing to do with making babies (but are, nevertheless, vital to staying alive). In addition to your ***bladder***, other non-reproductive organs include your ***intestines***, which carry digesting food along until waste material is ready to exit your body through your ***anus*** at the end of your ***rectum***.

Collectively, all the reproductive organs, and the non-reproductive organs, within your pelvic cavity are referred to as your ***pelvic organs***.

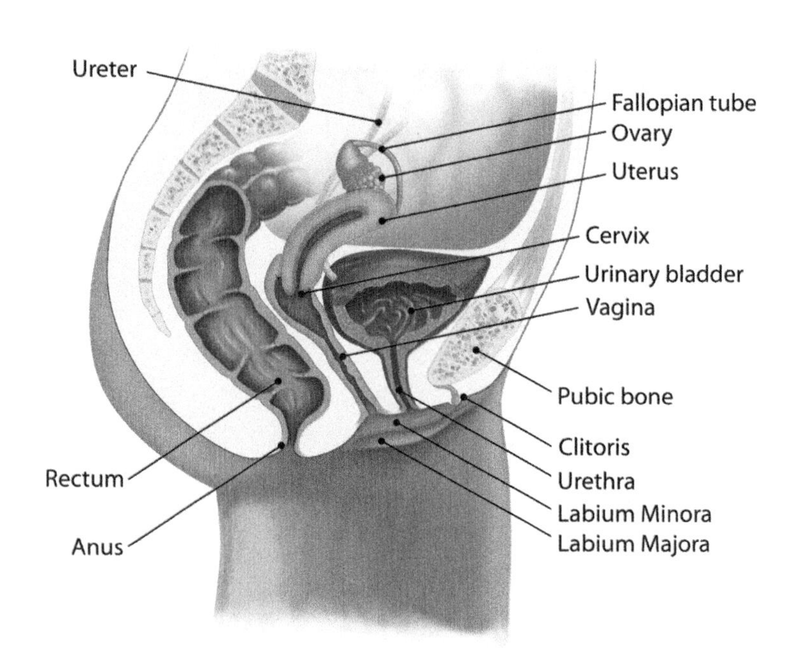

Hold Everything!

Pelvic Floor

Nature provided for your pelvic organs to be held in place by a strong muscular membrane at the bottom of your abdomen, which attaches to your pelvis. This region, quite aptly, is called your ***pelvic floor***.

Fascia

Muscles on the pelvic floor are responsible for tightly and firmly holding your vagina in its elevated position. Sheets of connective tissue, called ***fascia***, and ligaments also help support your pelvic organs by tying them in place.

Glossary of Terms

andropause. Male menopause. The time in a man's life characterized by a slow and steady decrease in the amount of testosterone in the system.

anus. Opening at the end of the rectum through which waste material exits the body.

apex. The top of the vaginal tube.

atrophy. Withering or wasting away of tissue, organ or part of the body.

Atypical Squamous Cells of Undetermined Significance (ASC-US). A common abnormal Pap test finding in which the cells look abnormal, but it is not known whether the abnormality is significant.

benign. Not dangerous.

Big Pharma. Common term for large pharmaceutical companies.

bioidentical hormones. Hormones with a molecular structure identical to the natural female sex hormones that the body already makes, or used to make before menopause.

bioidentical. A substance with a molecular structure that is identical to a substance that the body naturally produces.

birth canal. The passageway through which a baby travels as it is born.

bladder prolapse. Condition where the bladder drops out of its natural place inside the pelvic area.

bladder. Body organ for storing urine.

camel toe. When clothing rides up so tight between the legs that it creates a crack up the middle of the genitals.

carcinoma *in situ*. Stage that is one step away from cancer.

cervix. The medical term for the lower, narrow end of the uterus.

chlamydia. A sexually transmitted disease.

clitoris. The small sexual organ at the top of the vaginal opening.

collagen. A fibrous protein found in skin and other connective tissue.

colpocleisis. A surgical procedure that permanently closes the inside walls of the vagina.

colposcope. Instrument named from root words colpos (vagina) and scope (view).

colposcopy. A diagnostic test using a colposcope to view the vagina.

compounded prescriptions. Prescriptions made to order for each patient.

compounding pharmacies. Specialty pharmacies that make up custom preparations based on formulas prescribed by physicians.

conjugated. Formed by a union of compounds.

continence. The ability to hold urine in the bladder and control urine flow.

cystocele. The medical term for bulging of the bladder into the vagina.

cystourethrocele. Term for a cystocele and urethrocele occurring in combination.

endometriosis. A condition in which endometrial tissue is present in the ovaries or elsewhere in the body.

enterocele. Prolapse of the small intestine.

episiotomy. An incision to enlarge the opening to the vagina.

estradiol (E_2). A form of hormone present in the ovaries and the dominant estrogen in the body prior to menopause.

estriol (E_3). The estrogen produced during pregnancy.

estrogen. A woman's defining natural female sex hormone (produced in a woman's body in several forms), responsible for ovulation, menstrual periods, pregnancy, and for influencing essential body functions.

estrone ($E_{1.}$). The dominant form of estrogen in women after menopause, and in men.

excised. Surgically removed by cutting away.

fallopian tubes. Tubes extending from the uterus to the ovary that carry eggs and sperm, and where fertilization of the egg, or ovum, takes place.

fascia. Sheets of connective tissue.

fecal incontinence. To lose control of the bowel.

female circumcision. Removal of the small sexual organ at the top of the vaginal opening.

genitals. Visible external parts of the sex organs.

gonorrhea. A sexually transmitted disease.

GYN. Abbreviation for gynecology.

gynecology. The branch of medicine that deals with women's health, especially involving women's reproductive health.

high-risk human papilloma virus (HRHPV). A virus that can cause genital warts and that can lead to cervical cancer.

Hormone Hoop-La. Term describing the controversy resulting from the 2002 conclusions of a government study on heart disease conducted by the *Women's Health Initiative.*

human papilloma virus (HPV). A common virus that infects skin cells.

hymen. Thin, crescent-shaped membrane that partially covers the external vaginal opening.

hysterectomy. Removal of the uterus.

incontinence. Difficulty controlling the start and stop of urine flow or fecal material.

intestines. Non-reproductive pelvic organs that carry digesting food.

introitus. The small chamber just inside the vaginal opening.

Kegels. A set of vaginal squeezing exercises developed by Dr. Kegel.

labia majora. Two rounded folds of the vulva, composed of fatty tissue with slightly darker-colored skin along the outer surfaces.

labia minora. Two flat, reddish, inner tissue folds of the vulva, commonly referred to as "lips."

labia. The outer folds of the vulva that surround a woman's genital organs.

labial hypertrophy. The medical term for overgrowth of the labia.

labial reduction. A cosmetic surgery procedure for altering the inner and outer lips (folds of skin) surrounding a woman's vulva.

labiaplasty. Another term for labial reduction (alternately spelled labioplasty).

Laser Vaginal Rejuvenation (LVR). A process patented by Dr. David Matlock employing laser surgery.

LEEP. Abbreviation for loop electrosurgical excision procedure which removes abnormal tissue by cutting it away with a thin wire loop that carries an electrical current.

libido. Overall sexual drive.

Magnetic Resonance Imaging (MRI). A test that uses a magnetic field and pulses of radio wave energy to make pictures of organs.

menopause. The time in a woman's life when lack of natural hormones causes menstruation to cease, usually around age fifty-two.

metabolism. The efficient conversion of food into energy and other products the body needs to sustain life.

non-bioidentical hormones. Hormonal substances with a chemical composition not identical to hormones produced by the human body.

OB. Abbreviation for obstetrics.

obstetrics. The branch of medicine that deals with giving care to pregnant women and delivering babies.

off label. When physicians prescribe a drug for use in a different way than the FDA-approved drug label.

ovaries. Female reproductive organs that produce ovum.

ovum. Tiny reproductive cells also called eggs.

palpation. A medical term for examination using gentle pressure of the fingers to check for abnormalities.

Pap test. The common term for the Papanicolaou test, used to detect cervical cancer early.

pelvic floor. A strong muscular membrane at the bottom of the abdomen, which attaches to the pelvis.

pelvic organ prolapse. When pelvic organs, such as the bladder or rectum, drop down so that they bulge or protrude into the vaginal wall.

pelvic organs. Collectively, all the reproductive organs and the non-reproductive organs within the pelvic cavity.

pelvic support defects. Another term for pelvic organ prolapse.

perimenopause. The time before actual menopause when natural hormone production begins to diminish.

perineal area. The surface region between the vagina and the anus.

perineal body. The muscular area outside the bottom of the vaginal opening.

pessaries. Devices placed inside the vagina to mechanically push up or hold up prolapsing tissue.

pH balance. A measure of acid or base quality.

pharmaceutical prescriptions. Prescriptions that can be filled at local pharmacies.

postmenopause. The time in a woman's life after her ovaries are no longer functional and she has stopped having menstrual periods.

precancer. Abnormal cells that are not normal, but they are not yet cancer.

Premarin. A non-bioidentical hormone marketed by a leading drug company.

procidentia. The complete falling down of an organ from its normal anatomical position.

progesterone. The natural female sex hormone that acts within the womb and placenta in connection with pregnancy.

progestin. The version of progesterone synthesized by drug companies.

prolapse. "To drop" or "to sink." When one of the body organs drops out of its natural place inside the pelvic area.

Provera. A non-bioidentical form of progestin marketed by a leading drug company.

pudendal nerve. One of the pelvic nerves.

rectal prolapse. When the bowel bulges into the vagina.

rectocele. The medical term for the rectum bulging into or out of the vaginal wall.

rectum. The last part of the digestive tract.

rugation. Fold in a body part.

sling procedure. Procedure in which a surgeon implants a piece of material under the urethra to support it.

stress urinary incontinence. Inability to control bursts of urine.

synthesized. Produced by a chemical process.

testosterone. A male steroid hormone produced in men's testicles, also made in smaller quantities by women in ovaries and adrenal glands.

thyroid. A butterfly-shaped gland situated between and just above the collar bones.

tibial nerve stimulation. A treatment that helps with constant pangs of urinary urgency.

urethra. The tube that carries urine out of the body.

urethrocele. When the urethra bulges into the vaginal wall.

urgency incontinence. A continual urge to urinate.

urinary incontinence. Difficulty controlling the start and stop of urine flow.

uterine prolapse. When the uterus drops down into the vagina.

uterus. The richly-lined cavity where a baby develops and obtains nourishment during pregnancy.

vagina. A hollow tube about three to seven inches long, forming a pathway from a woman's uterus to outside her body.

vaginal dilators. Firm rubber inserts in sets that progress larger in diameter, used to gradually dilate or stretch the vagina back to a normal width and depth.

vaginal mucosa. Tissue within the vagina.

vaginal opening. The outer opening of the vagina.

Vaginal Regenalift™. Trademarked procedure in which the surgeon injects platelet-rich-plasma along suture lines to promote rapid healing.

vaginal vault prolapse. When the top of the vagina bulges down into the lower vagina.

vulva. The external female genitalia, visible from outside, surrounding the vaginal opening.

To contact Dr. King, click the “Contact Me” tab on her website:
http://www.DrGailKing.com

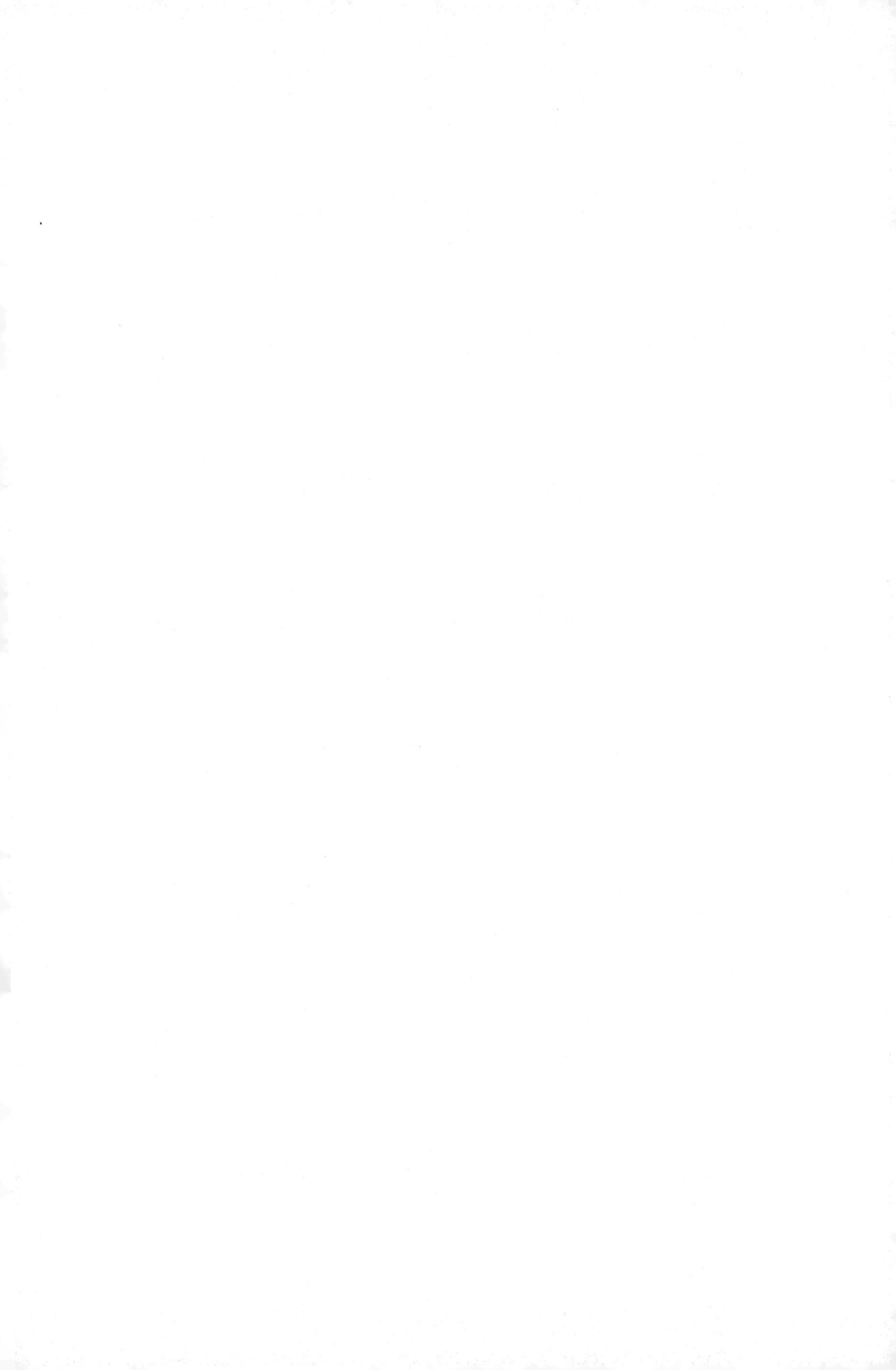

CPSIA information can be obtained
at www.ICGtesting.com
Printed in the USA
LVOW05s1005281215
468072LV00002B/2/P